THE 28-DAY DASH DIET
WEIGHT-LOSS PROGRAM

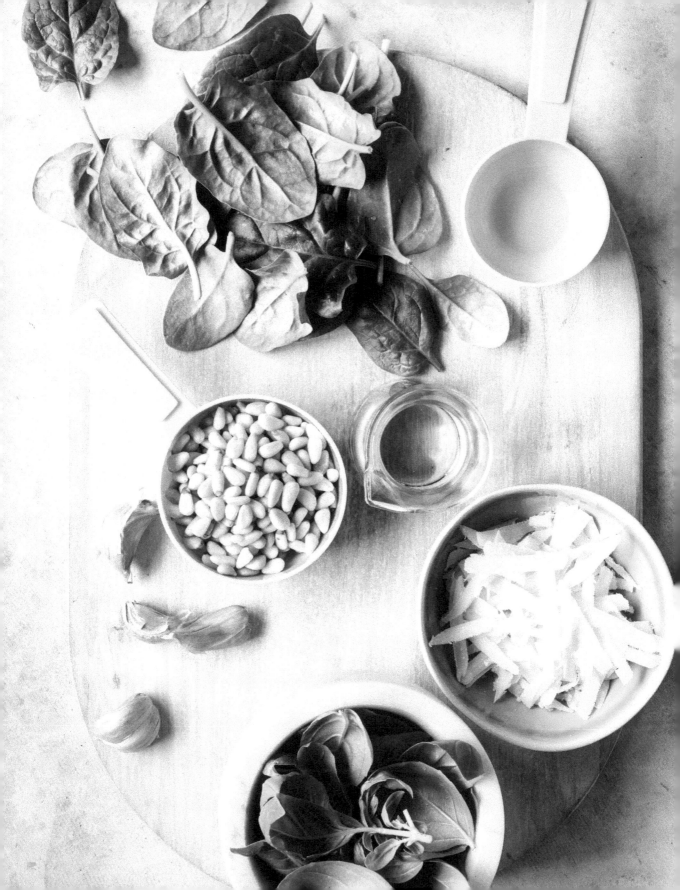

THE 28-DAY

DASH Diet

WEIGHT-LOSS PROGRAM

Recipes and Workouts to Lower
Blood Pressure and Improve Your Health

**ANDY DE SANTIS, RD, MPH, and
JULIE ANDREWS, MS, RDN, CD**

FOREWORD BY ANNIE F. KELLY, MD, FACC

Photography by Nadine Greeff

**ROCKRIDGE
PRESS**

For general information on our other products and services or to obtain technical support, please contact our Customer Care Department within the United States at (866) 744-2665, or outside the United States at (510) 253-0500.

Rockridge Press publishes its books in a variety of electronic and print formats. Some content that appears in print may not be available in electronic books, and vice versa.

TRADEMARKS: Rockridge Press and the Rockridge Press logo are trademarks or registered trademarks of Callisto Media Inc. and/or its affiliates, in the United States and other countries, and may not be used without written permission. All other trademarks are the property of their respective owners. Rockridge Press is not associated with any product or vendor mentioned in this book.

Interior Designer: Liz Cosgrove & Meg Woodcheke
Cover Designer: Amy King
Editor: Salwa Jabado
Production Editor: Andrew Yackira
Photography: © 2018 Nadine Greeff
Illustrations: © 2018 Charlie Layton

ISBN: Print 978-1-64152-139-0 | eBook 978-1-64152-140-6

We would like to sincerely thank you for including
us on your journey to better health. We take this responsibility very
seriously, and have worked diligently to ensure that this book is
everything that you hope and expect it to be.

CHICKPEA CAULIFLOWER TIKKA MASALA,
page 132

Contents

Foreword

Heart disease currently remains the number one killer in men and women. Now more than ever, the medical community is caring for patients in a multifaceted and multidisciplinary fashion, with teams of subspecialized cardiologists. Interventionalists, echocardiographers, cardiothoracic surgeons, electrophysiologists, and heart failure specialists are all working together to provide the most optimal care for each individual patient. However, dietary interventions, which are so meaningful, often get short shrift.

I first met Julie Andrews during her time as lead dietitian of the Learning Kitchen, which was co-located with my clinic. Julie kindly extended an invitation to me for her "Heart Healthy Cooking" class. As I stood in class for the first time in front of a stainless-steel table with culinary devices (many which I found unfamiliar), I secretly thought to myself: As a physician, I universally recommended the DASH diet, quoting the many benefits. In reality, however, I offered little on how to actually execute the dietary changes. Julie started off the class with knife skills, introduced us to the tools, and then we had fun, making salmon with pesto, immersion blending butternut squash soup, and preparing blueberry crumble. It was healthy, educational, and fit within the DASH diet prescriptive.

This experience changed how I coached my patients. It was ineffective to simply dictate recommendations. There had to be active engagement—identifying and overcoming barriers, and guiding them to design their own SMART goals. This is exactly what you'll find in *The 28-Day DASH Diet Weight-Loss Program*.

After a heart attack, our patients now participate in cardiac rehabilitation working closely with exercise physiologists and dietitians. Establishing routine exercise habits and healthy eating patterns is the key, and hard to execute alone. My favorite recommendations include using smartphone applications to track exercise and tally nutritional intake, meeting with registered dietitians who work alongside us in clinic or within our community grocery stores, mindfulness meditation, and participating in Community Supported Agriculture (often reimbursable with health insurance). I've now added *The 28-Day DASH Diet Weight-Loss Program* to my list of recommendations.

Andy De Santis and Julie Andrews have thoughtfully provided the evidence behind the DASH diet and laid out a 28-day menu and exercise plan. This eliminates half the work of meal prep, immediately answers the daily "What's for dinner?" question, and allows you to have fun in the kitchen.

As a working mom with 3 young children, family dinners are important to me. The challenge I face every day is preparing a fresh meal that is timely, with ingredients that are actually in my fridge that everyone will enjoy, with leftovers that will actually be eaten or repurposed into another delicious meal.

Welcome, and thank you for joining me on this 28-day DASH diet journey, forming sustainable healthier habits for you and your family. This book is not about what you cannot do. It is all about what you can do.

Annie F. Kelly, MD, FACC
Associate Professor
Director, Outpatient Cardiovascular Medicine Services
Division of Cardiovascular Medicine
University of Wisconsin-Madison

Introduction

My clients have the same concerns that you do—they are worried about their weight, their blood pressure, and their diet and health. As a registered dietitian who operates a private practice centered on healthy eating, chronic disease risk reduction, and weight management, believe me when I say that when it comes to diets, I've seen them all. Low carb, high carb, low fat, high protein, and others. As different as they may appear on the surface, these diets are characterized by similar issues. They are extremely restrictive, they are difficult to maintain, and they ignore overall wellness. Although they may help some people lose weight in the short term, their long-term success rates are limited.

You should know right off the bat it won't be like that here. DASH (Dietary Approaches to Stop Hypertension) is simply different. As you will see in this book, it is not about unpleasant restrictions, quick fixes, or extreme short-term changes. *The 28-Day DASH Diet Weight-Loss Program* uses a comprehensive approach to help you lower blood pressure, lose weight, and achieve positive long-term health benefits. I have helped hundreds of clients understand how changing the way they eat can enhance their health and quality of life and I can help you, too. I'd like to think of our DASH diet program as the first 28 days of the rest of your life. It's a diet in name only, because it is not about what you *can't* eat—it instead focuses on the inclusion of a wide variety of foods, including fruits, vegetables, whole grains, nuts, seeds, low-fat meat and dairy, and—yes–oils and sweets, too. All of the things you would want and expect to eat are exactly what the DASH diet offers. For this reason, the DASH style of eating really does offer people a pathway to sustained success not only in terms of improving

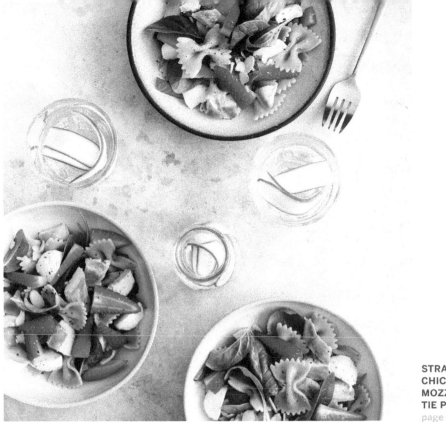

STRAWBERRY, CHICKEN & MOZZARELLA BOW TIE PASTA SALAD, page 106

their dietary adequacy and lowering their blood pressure but in terms of losing weight as well.

One of the important things that I want you to understand before we go any further is there is no such thing as a one-size-fits-all solution when it comes to healthy eating. I am going to teach you everything you ever wanted to know about the DASH diet in combination with a host of other guidance to help you move toward a healthier lifestyle. I draw on a combination of scientific evidence and my own experience in private practice to offer tips, tricks, and practical solutions to provide you every opportunity for success. If you bring to the table a desire for lifestyle change, I am confident that I can help get you closer to where you want to be.

In addition to the dietary guidance, this book covers other important aspects of good health including exercise, sleep, and stress management. We have included a practical and actionable 28-day program that puts all of this knowledge to work in a structured way. It is anchored by 100 unique, delicious, and nutritious recipes curated by my colleague and coauthor, Julie Andrews. Let's get started learning more about the DASH diet.

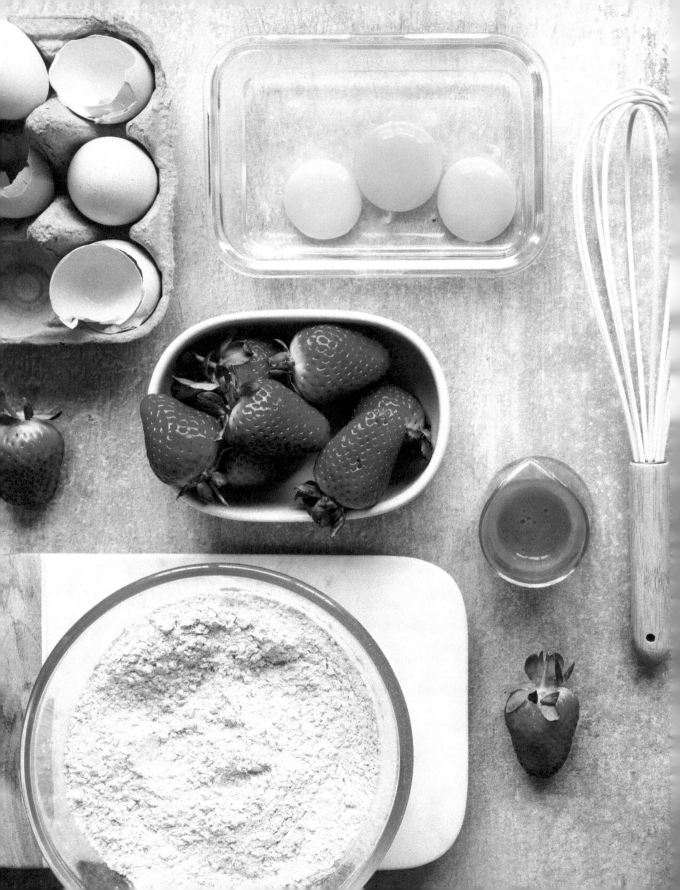

PART ONE

Getting Started

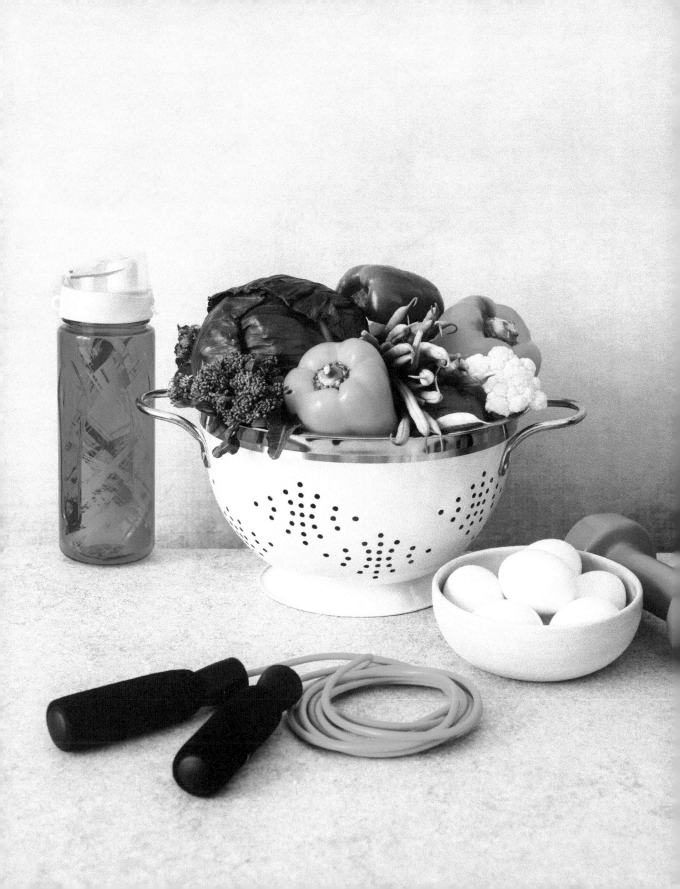

Your
DASH Diet Primer

The DASH diet represents a balanced, varied style of eating that offers you a practical nutrition solution to help you move toward your goals. Healthy eating is complicated by all of the fad diets and trends in the world. We are going to ignore that and focus on a style of eating that you can really feel confident in. Here, we will take a closer look at why the DASH diet is so different, and so much better, than what you may be used to.

From the Standard American Diet to the DASH Diet

The average American's diet needs some improvement. Health concerns such as obesity, diabetes, and hypertension have become more of a norm than an exception. According to the 2013–2014 data from the National Health and Nutrition Examination Survey, more than two-thirds of the American population was considered either overweight or obese. This is partially due to a disconnect between the amount of calories we consume from food, the amount our bodies need, and the amount we expend through physical activity. What's much more concerning is the reality that approximately one in three American adults has high blood pressure, also known as hypertension, which is one of the most significant risk factors for cardiovascular disease. This does not even mention the fact that so few of us consume adequate amounts of the most healthful foods like fruits and vegetables.

This is where the Dietary Approaches to Stop Hypertension (DASH) eating style, which was developed and tested specifically with the purpose of addressing the pervasive issue of high blood pressure, or hypertension, comes in. First unveiled in an article in *The New England Journal of Medicine* in 1997, the DASH diet has grown in mainstream popularity, and was ranked as the number one Best Diet for Healthy Eating by the *U.S. News & World Report* in 2018, which also ranked it number four on the list of easiest diets to follow.

The ultimate goal of this chapter is to introduce you to the DASH diet and help you understand how, in combination with a holistic approach to a healthy lifestyle, it can put you on the path to lower blood pressure and improved cardiovascular health while also supporting your weight-loss goals.

How DASH Diet Aids in Weight Loss and Lowers Blood Pressure

The DASH diet is highlighted by its inclusion of ample fruits, vegetables, and low-fat dairy products while also being generally low in saturated fat. The blood pressure lowering qualities of the DASH diet are often attributed to it being naturally high in potassium, calcium, and magnesium, which are found abundantly in the diverse array of foods that the diet incorporates.

In 2001, the DASH group conducted a follow-up study to the one published in 1997 and again published their results in *The New England Journal of Medicine*. The study found the DASH diet was even more effective at lowering blood pressure when combined with dietary sodium restriction. Excessive sodium, or salt, intake has since become well known to increase some people's risk for hypertension. Changes to diet while also restricting sodium has become recognized as effective to lower blood pressure. These DASH diet trials, and a number of others that followed, effectively proved that the DASH diet can significantly reduce your blood pressure.

But how does the DASH dietary pattern stack up for those who may be trying to lose weight? From my perspective as a registered dietitian, the DASH diet offers you the opportunity to shed unwanted pounds in a practical and nonrestrictive way. For example, the DASH diet contains plenty of fruits and whole grains, which many common diets restrict. It focuses on balanced and moderate inclusion of all different types of foods. With that in mind, it comes as no surprise that a 2016 review study published in the *Obesity Reviews* journal concluded that the "DASH diet is a good choice for weight management, particularly for weight reduction in overweight and obese participants."

Caloric Intake on the DASH Diet

The DASH diet guidelines center on the inclusion of a wide variety of food groups in amounts that vary based on individual characteristics. These food groups and their recommended serving sizes are determined by personal characteristics including your age, gender, and activity level. Before you can determine your own personal DASH diet guidelines, you need to estimate your calorie needs. The first two tables below will help you estimate your body's daily caloric needs. In order to figure out your estimated daily calorie intake, take a look at your physical activity. **Sedentary** is defined as little to no physical activity, **moderately active** as walking 1½ to 3 miles a day plus light physical activity, and **active** as exercising at the level suggested by the 28-day plan that follows.

Estimated Daily Calorie Needs for Women

AGE (YEARS)	SEDENTARY	MODERATELY ACTIVE	ACTIVE
19–30	2,000	2,100	2,400
31–50	1,800	2,000	2,200
51+	1,600	1,800	2,100

Estimated Daily Calorie Needs for Men

AGE (YEARS)	SEDENTARY	MODERATELY ACTIVE	ACTIVE
19–30	2,400	2,700	3,000
31–50	2,200	2,500	2,900
51+	2,000	2,300	2,600

Keep in mind that if your goal is to reduce your body weight, a simple first step is to consume approximately 250 to 500 calories fewer than what the above tables estimate. Please consult the charts below, which you can then use with the Daily Serving Recommendations table (page 19) to determine your approximate serving recommendations for each food group. With that in mind, I want you to worry less about the actual number of calories you are aiming for and more about what this means in terms of total daily servings in the DASH diet.

Estimated Daily Calorie Needs for Women Who Want to Lose Weight

AGE (YEARS)	SEDENTARY	MODERATELY ACTIVE	ACTIVE
19–30	1,500–1,750	1,600–1,850	1,900–2,150
31–50	1,300–1,550	1,500–1,750	1,700–1,950
51+	1,100–1,350	1,300–1,550	1,600–1,850

Estimated Daily Calorie Needs for Men Who Want to Lose Weight

AGE (YEARS)	SEDENTARY	MODERATELY ACTIVE	ACTIVE
19–30	1,900-2,150	2,200–2,450	2,500–2,750
31–50	1,700-1,950	2,000–2,250	2,400–2,650
51+	1,500-1,750	1,800–2,050	2,100–2,350

The DASH Diet Guidelines

It is important to identify the different kinds of foods that the DASH diet encourages you to consume. There are some general guidelines to eating in a DASH-friendly way. Simply put, you should eat more fruits, vegetables, low-fat dairy foods, whole grains, fish, poultry, and nuts. You should cut back on foods that are high in saturated fat, cholesterol, and trans fats. You should limit the amount of sodium, sweets, sugary drinks, and red meat that you consume. But how and why? Let's discuss the different kinds of foods you should be consuming and why they help improve your health.

WHOLE GRAINS AND STARCHY VEGETABLES

Let's face it: Almost all of us love carbohydrate-rich foods, and although very-low-carb diets may help some lose weight in the short term, they aren't particularly sustainable and certainly not very enjoyable. The DASH diet doesn't suggest avoiding carbs; it suggests you enjoy the most fiber- and nutrient-dense versions of them, which is a message I can certainly get behind. Brown rice, quinoa, whole-grain bread, whole-grain pasta, and potatoes (any variety) are DASH-approved.

Serving size: 1 slice whole-grain bread, ½ cup brown rice or quinoa, 1 medium-size potato or sweet potato.

VEGETABLES

Vegetables are, simply put, the most important part of any eating style. The high potassium content of most vegetables—especially leafy greens—plays an important role in blood pressure regulation. Your kidneys play an important role in blood pressure management by controlling the fluid balance in your body. This balance is further modified by your sodium and potassium intake. Most people consume much more sodium than potassium, which affects your kidneys' ability to properly control your blood pressure. This balance can be restored in most people by increasing potassium intake and decreasing sodium intake. Vegetables contain a vast amount of other healthful nutrients and antioxidant compounds. From a weight-management perspective, the high fiber content of vegetables promotes satiety and may prevent weight gain. A 2009 study in *The Journal of Nutrition* found that women who increased their fiber intake tended to gain less weight and body fat over time. Most Americans simply do not eat enough fiber, with only about half the population consuming the American Heart Association's recommended daily target goal of 30 grams per day.

Serving size: ½ cup cooked veggies like broccoli or Brussels sprouts, 1 cup raw vegetables like spinach.

FRUIT

Sometimes popular "diets" suggest eliminating fruit because it contains moderate amounts of natural sugars. If this is something you've heard, I want you to ignore that sentiment and embrace fruit as a very healthy component of the DASH diet and a critical part of longevity and good health. Fruit, aside from being absolutely delicious, is rich in potassium, fiber, and other important nutrients that help support both blood pressure and weight management.

Serving size: 1 medium-size piece of fruit like an apple or banana, ½ cup fruit like blueberries or strawberries.

LOW-FAT DAIRY AND ALTERNATIVES

Dairy products and alternatives are an important part of the DASH eating plan for a few reasons. The high calcium content of these foods is thought to play an important role in blood-pressure regulation because it modifies the hormones that are responsible for the tension in your blood vessels. The high protein content also supports weight management and weight loss, because protein not only makes us feel full but requires extra energy for our bodies to break down. This largely explains why studies, including a 2015 review published in *The American Journal of Clinical Nutrition*, tend to find that adequate protein intake is usually associated with better outcomes when it comes to managing both our weight and our appetite.

Serving size: 1 cup skim milk, 1 cup 0% yogurt (including Greek), 1 cup soy milk, 1½ ounces skim cheese.

LEAN MEAT, POULTRY, FISH, AND ALTERNATIVES

These are dietary staples for many and important contributors of protein and magnesium in the DASH diet. For anyone who happens to be vegan or vegetarian, know that you can confidently replace animal-protein sources listed here with legume-based protein such as tofu, lentils, chickpeas, and others. When selecting meat, leaner cuts like tenderloin, sirloin, or eye of round for beef are optimal as they contain less fat than other commonly available varieties. Avoiding purchasing cuts with visible fat or trimming fat before cooking also helps. We suggest consuming multiple servings of fish per week.

Serving size: 1 ounce of cooked meat, poultry, or fish, 1 egg, 3 ounces of tofu

NUTS, SEEDS, AND LEGUMES

This group of foods is unique for the simple fact they are among the relatively small group of plant-based foods that contain both iron and protein, which are two of the important nutrients animal proteins offer us. Unlike most types of meat, though, these choices are high in fiber and heart-healthy monounsaturated fat while also being much lower in saturated fat.

Serving size: ⅓ cup raw or unsalted nuts or seeds, 2 tablespoons nut butter, ½ cup cooked legumes (preferably cooked from raw, not canned, which are higher in sodium).

HEALTHY FATS AND OILS

This group contains the types of foods we might either top food with or use to cook with. When people think of healthy fats, they often think about olive oil and other vegetable oils, which are a great choice and certainly better choices than the likes of lard or butter. Even so, it's important to be mindful of how much of these items we use because, in addition to being calorie-dense, many of the nutritional benefits of oils are offered in greater supply in foods like nuts and seeds, which also keep us feeling full due to their fiber content. We suggest making your own salad dressing out of oil and vinegar. If choosing store-bought, opt for the refrigerated versions, and be sure to read the labels and choose the lowest sodium version. We also offer salad dressing recipes that are better for you in our recipe section.

Serving size: 1 teaspoon oil, 2 tablespoons light salad dressing, 1 tablespoon standard dressing.

MORE ON OILS FROM CHEF JULIE

We want the majority of our fat intake from oils to come from unsaturated fats while a little can come from saturated. It is recommended to avoid trans fats, also known as hydrogenated oils. Depending on the type of fatty acids in oils and how they were processed, each has a unique smoke point or burn point, meaning different oils should be used for different applications.

- When cooking with high heat, such as roasting, stir-frying, or grilling, use neutral unsaturated oils, such as canola or avocado oil. Canola is relatively inexpensive yet contains omega-3 fatty acids. Avocado is also a great choice, as it's primarily made up of monounsaturated fatty acids and has the highest smoke point of all oils, but it's also a bit more expensive. They are both excellent cooking oils; it just depends on your personal choice and budget. For most of the recipes in this book, these oils are appropriate. I put "canola oil" in the recipes because it is the least expensive option, but feel free to use whichever one you prefer. If you are trying to avoid genetically modified organisms (GMOs), choose organic canola oil, as any food item that is labeled organic has to also be free of GMOs by law.

- When cooking with low heat, such as a quick sauté, or when making most salad dressings, use extra-virgin olive oil, which is also high in monounsaturated fats. It has a low smoke point, so it's best not to roast, stir-fry, or grill with it at high temperatures.

When an oil starts to burn, the chemical composition changes, and it may no longer be a healthy option. Other olive oils, like extra light, have been processed differently and have a higher smoke point. These are also great oils to use in higher-heat cooking if you prefer the olive oil flavor. I enjoy using olive oils for recipes that are Mediterranean-style, as the flavor lends itself well to those dishes. In this book, you will see olive oil indicated where it is most appropriate.

There are many other oils on the market, and the ones I've mentioned above aren't the only nutritious options. We've chosen a handful of oils we regularly use because of their nutritional properties and cooking applications and have shared them with you to keep things simple and affordable.

Due to its recent popularity, we should also discuss coconut oil. The studies on it are mixed, given that it's a saturated fat but also a plant, so we generally recommend consuming it occasionally, such as when making a granola bar recipe or when baking.

SWEETS

The final proof that the DASH diet is quite unlike any diet you've probably tried before is that you can have dessert. Yes, you can have sweets, and—yes—you can have them more than just once a week. The unfortunate reality is that for many people, diets are difficult to maintain because of their restrictive nature. The DASH plan is a long-term sustainable eating style that promotes enjoying both food and life. Don't worry, you can still have ice cream in moderation.

> **Serving size:** ½ cup ice cream or frozen yogurt; 1 tablespoon syrup, honey, or sugar; 1 cup juice or other sugar-sweetened drink.

SODIUM

Sodium, which is commonly known as the salt we find in or add to food, is often overconsumed and one of the key drivers of high blood pressure. Specific strategies on how to consume sodium within the 2,300-milligram daily limit will be discussed at length below.

> **Goal:** Under 2,300 milligrams daily to start (1 teaspoon), working toward a maximum 1,500 milligrams (¾ teaspoon) daily.

LOWER-SODIUM LIVING

In some people, prolonged excessive sodium intake contributes to high blood pressure partially because it can lead to chronic fluid retention, which ultimately strains your blood vessels. However, cutting the amount of salt in your diet may not be as simple as just putting away the shaker. It will, in fact, take a multifaceted approach for most people to make a significant dent in their daily intake. Let's take a closer look at the three areas where you can do this most effectively:

At the grocery store: Your mission to reduce the amount of sodium in your diet starts at the grocery store. Any food product sold in a box or a bottle, ranging from crackers to pasta sauces, could potentially have a very high sodium content. Your best defense is utilizing the labels on these products to compare sodium content among similar foods in the same category. Choosing the product that is lowest in sodium is a great first step.

At home: Did you know that a single teaspoon of salt contains your DASH diet sodium limit (2,300 milligrams) for the day? Those who don't add salt to their food won't be concerned by this, but if you are a heavy user it may be time to consider relying on herbs, spices, or sodium-free blends of both. When you use them in combination with acidic flavors such as those offered by lemon juice or vinegar, you won't miss a thing from a taste perspective and will ultimately need to rely less on sodium-heavy condiments from the grocery store. And the best part: There are 100 delicious lower-sodium recipes waiting for you in part 2 (page 75) of this book.

Eating out: Any given meal purchased out, as compared to made at home, is likely to have significantly higher sodium content. This is problematic for those living with high blood pressure and especially true of selections that are heavy in sauces, such as pasta dishes. Other heavily salted restaurant items might include French fries or various soup dishes. For this reason, setting goals around how many meals you purchase out a week is an important part of your lifestyle going forward.

Kick-Start Your DASH Diet Weight-Loss Program

Up until this point I've guided you through the basics of the DASH diet while also identifying how and why it can be your secret to healthy eating success. But the learning doesn't stop here. As we progress together through this book, more of your questions about balanced eating, calories, exercise, and meal planning will be answered.

You will not only learn about the DASH diet but also find out how to seamlessly incorporate its principles into your daily life to offer you a lasting, long-term solution to your health concerns. I know weight loss is at the top of your mind, so we will take the next steps in this journey by more closely discussing why weight loss can be such a challenge and how you can make the most of the inclusivity of the DASH diet to overcome many of the struggles you may have encountered in the past with restrictive diets.

From there, I will lead you into a discussion of all the other important components of your holistic approach to health, including strategies for improved sleep, exercise, and stress management, all of which will help you make the most of what the DASH diet has to offer.

You are, above all else, going to learn how to improve the way you eat using fun and delicious recipes. The 28-day plan that is still to come will allow you to effortlessly incorporate the DASH diet principles into your daily life and set you on the path toward long-term success.

It all starts now.

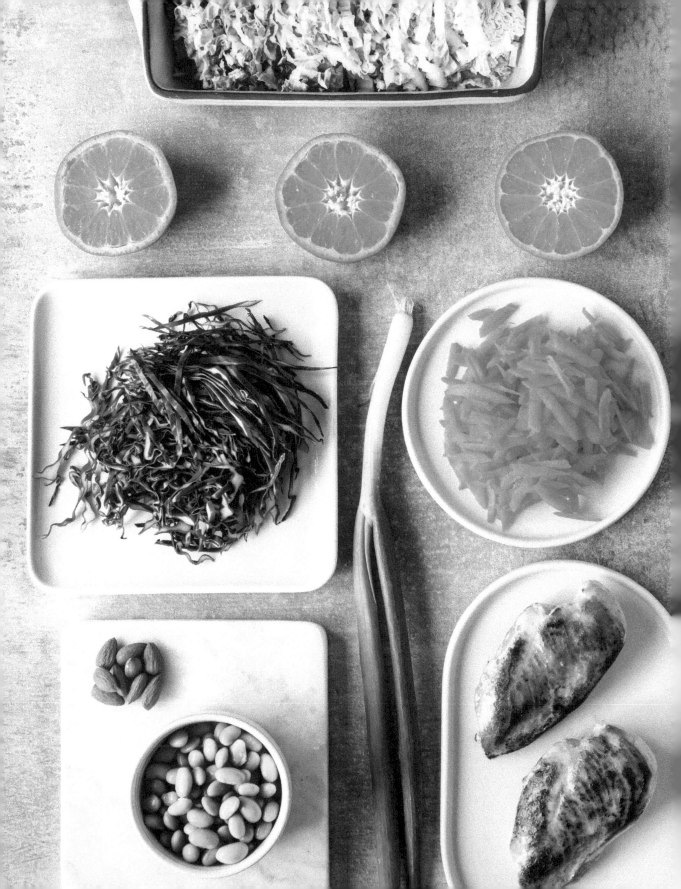

Tackling Weight Loss

The best part of the DASH diet is that it can offer you a path to weight loss that is rooted in healthy, balanced eating. With that being said, weight loss is a challenge, and maintaining weight loss is an even bigger one. Part of the reason why many people may struggle to lose weight or keep it off is that they may rely on unsustainable dietary patterns. Fortunately, one of the major strengths of the DASH diet is that it is a sustainable, unrestrictive, and relatively easy-to-follow way to successfully manage your weight. In this section, we will learn more about the science behind weight loss, and practical strategies to manage your expectations and improve your chances of success.

Understanding Calories

Calories represent the amount of energy found in food. Your body requires this energy at the cellular level to carry out molecular tasks but also to fuel the physical tasks of everyday life. A general rule of thumb: If you eat more calories than your body needs, you may gain weight over time. The opposite may occur if you eat less than you need. There's a lot more to it than that, though. Your genetics, hormones, metabolism, and physical activity level will also play an important role in determining how your body weight interacts with your food and calorie intake.

What ultimately happens to so many of us is that we chronically consume more calories than our bodies need while also living a relatively sedentary lifestyle that involves minimal caloric expenditure. This combination can result in a significant increase in body fat over time, particularly around the waist. Why does this matter? Well, the Centers for Disease Control (CDC) considers waist circumference a screening tool for disease risk. Men whose waist circumference is greater than 40 inches and nonpregnant women who have a waist circumference greater than 35 inches may be at greater risk of diabetes, high blood pressure, and cardiovascular disease.

Now let's consider the fact that one pound of body fat stores about 3,500 calories. Theoretically, if you are able to take in 500 calories less than your body requires each day to maintain its weight, you could expect to lose about 1 pound of fat a week (500 calories multiplied by 7 days equals 3,500 calories, or 1 pound of body fat). This theory offers a practical starting point for many people but also has limitations. For example, it does not account for the fact that as you lose weight, your metabolism will shift because a smaller body burns fewer calories. Although this is both an oversimplification and a generalization, it partially explains why weight loss slows down over time.

Regardless of changes to metabolism that occur with time, the primary initial goal of any legitimate weight-loss effort is to create what is known as a negative energy balance, which essentially just means taking in fewer calories than your body needs to maintain its current weight. A 2007 study from the *Annals of Nutrition and Metabolism* concluded that no matter what specific strategy or approach is used to attempt weight loss, a negative energy balance remains the most significant and primary driver. The main purpose of discussing these findings is to help you appreciate that calories and weight loss are complex, and we all respond to them differently.

Now that you know a bit more about how calories work, I'm going to ask you to put them aside. Yes, they are a relevant component of weight management, and I will be speaking about them again, but I don't want you to get overwhelmed or overly consumed by the concept of calories.

Calories are a singular characteristic of a food. They are not what make you feel full, satisfied, healthy, or happy. It's the type and amount of food that you eat that plays the much bigger role in determining those things. This is something that I don't want you to lose sight of as we move forward with our discussion. Next, you'll learn about the appropriate portions of food and see how many servings of food you should consume to meet your daily intake goals, which will make it easier to put calorie counting aside in favor of consuming the appropriate servings of a range of foods.

Portion Control

The most important part of the DASH diet is to eat healthy, nutrient-dense foods. The second most important part is to eat those wonderful foods with the appropriate frequency for your body's needs. There's absolutely no denying the fact that following the DASH diet principles, regardless of changes to your weight, will have a significant positive impact on your overall health and greatly benefit your blood pressure. However, when it comes to losing weight specifically, that extra bit of attention to portion sizes will allow you to enjoy the great diversity of foods available to you on the DASH eating plan while still putting you in a position to progress toward your weight-loss goals.

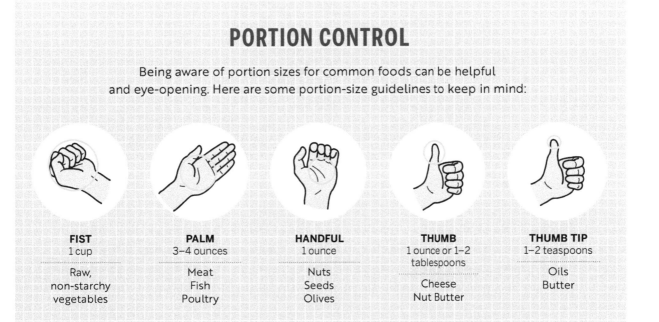

PORTION CONTROL

Being aware of portion sizes for common foods can be helpful and eye-opening. Here are some portion-size guidelines to keep in mind:

FIST	PALM	HANDFUL	THUMB	THUMB TIP
1 cup	3–4 ounces	1 ounce	1 ounce or 1–2 tablespoons	1–2 teaspoons
Raw, non-starchy vegetables	Meat Fish Poultry	Nuts Seeds Olives	Cheese Nut Butter	Oils Butter

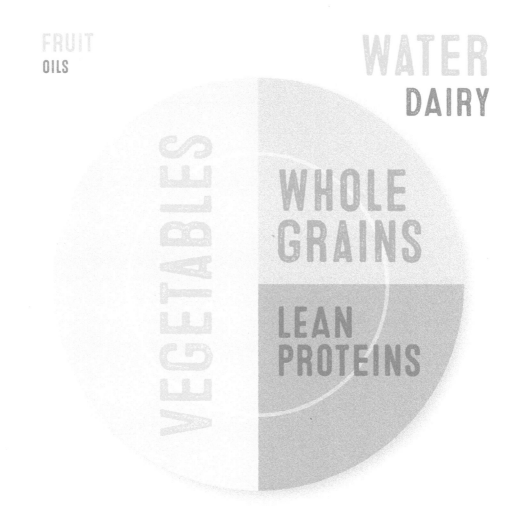

FRUIT
OILS

WATER
DAIRY

VEGETABLES

WHOLE GRAINS

LEAN PROTEINS

The healthy plate model above helps you understand what the ideal meal on the DASH diet looks like. The ultimate goal is to provide you with a guideline for meals that keeps you both full and nourished.

In the pillars of the DASH diet, fruits, vegetables, and starches such as whole grains all represent significant components. Each of these foods plays an important role in the blood-pressure-lowering and weight-management component of the diet, which is why they are all represented on the healthy plate. Vegetables should be the most significant portion of your meal because they help you feel full and nourished with a minimal intake of calories. Starches are represented by whole grains like brown rice or quinoa and also by starchy vegetable options like sweet potatoes. Fruit, which you can think of as a healthy post-meal treat, is represented by a piece of fruit like an apple or ½ cup fruit like berries or grapes. Protein plays an important role in both allowing you to feel satisfied and keeping your body strong. The role of protein can be filled by fish, lean poultry, or red meat as well as tofu. Keeping the oil usage for meal prep to around 1 tablespoon is a great way to manage calories, and using a piece of fruit as a sweet treat after your meal is another great choice.

IDENTIFYING YOUR FOOD SERVINGS BASED ON DAILY CALORIC INTAKE

Below you will find serving guidelines for a broad sample of calorie levels. Since exact calorie estimates vary widely from person to person, it's important to know that you can simply adjust your serving sizes according to the patterns observed in the table below. This will help you logically adjust your intake for higher and lower calorie levels. See the Estimated Daily Calorie Needs charts on page 5 to determine your calorie intake. Remember that consuming 250 to 500 calories below your needs in order to create a negative energy balance is a practical starting point to support weight loss. If your goal is losing weight, be sure to subtract 250 to 500 calories from your estimated calorie intake, or see the charts on page 6, with calorie intake for weight loss.

Daily Serving Recommendations

FOOD GROUP	CALORIE LEVEL				
	1,400	1,600	1,800	2,000	2,600
Grains	5–6 servings	6 servings	6 servings	6–8 servings	10–11 servings
Vegetables	3–4 servings	3–4 servings	4–5 servings	4–5 servings	5–6 servings
Fruit	4 servings	4 servings	4–5 servings	4–5 servings	5–6 servings
Dairy	2–3 servings	2–3 servings	2–3 servings	2–3 servings	3 servings
Meat, Poultry, Fish	3–4 servings	3–4 servings	4–6 servings	4–6 servings	6 servings
Nuts, Seeds, Legumes	3 servings per week	3–4 servings per week	4 servings per week	4–5 servings per week	1 serving per day
Fats and oils	1 serving	2 servings	2–3 servings	2–3 servings	3 servings
Sweets	3 servings per week	3 servings per week	5 servings per week	5 servings per week	1 serving per day
Sodium	Less than 2,300 mg	Less than 2,300 mg	Less than 2,300 mg	Less than 2,300 mg	Less than 2,300 mg

Serving size recommendations determined per National Institute of Health DASH guidelines.

Now that you have a better idea of how many servings you will require from each food group to meet your goals, fill out your own personal chart below based on your caloric needs, and take a closer look at the importance of each individual grouping and what a single serving size actually looks like.

FOOD GROUP	MY CALORIE LEVEL_____ MY NUMBER OF DAILY SERVINGS
Grains (1 serving = 1 slice whole grain bread, ½ cup brown rice or quinoa, 1 medium size potato or sweet potato)	
Vegetables (1 serving = ½ cup cooked veggies like broccoli or Brussels sprouts, 1 cup raw vegetables like spinach)	
Fruit (1 serving = 1 medium size piece of fruit like an apple or banana, ½ cup fruit like blueberries or strawberries)	
Dairy (1 serving = 1 cup skim milk; 1 cup 0% yogurt, including Greek; 1 cup soy milk; 1½ ounces skim cheese varieties)	
Meat, Poultry, Fish (1 serving = 1 ounce of cooked meat, poultry, or fish; 1 egg; 3 ounces of tofu)	
Nuts, Seeds, Legumes (1 serving = ⅓ cup raw or unsalted nuts or seeds, 2 tablespoons nut butter, ½ cup cooked legumes)	
Fats and oils (1 serving = 1 teaspoon oil or margarine, 2 tablespoons light salad dressing, 1 tablespoon standard dressing)	
Sweets (1 serving = ½ cup ice cream or frozen yogurt; 1 ounce chocolate; 1 cookie; 1 tablespoon syrup, honey, or sugar; 1 cup juice or other sugar-sweetened drink)	
Sodium (Under 2,300 milligrams daily to start [1 teaspoon], working toward a maximum 1,500 milligrams [¾ teaspoon] daily.)	

The menu plans offered in chapter 4 (page 45) of this book were created with the 1,600-calorie level in mind, which represents the estimated needs of women in the 51+ age category who are active and have a goal to lose weight. Those with higher or lower calorie needs can use the calorie-specific tables above to approximate and adjust their intake via increasing or decreasing their portion sizes at meals or incorporating extra snacks or side dishes, as provided in the recipe chapters, to meet their differing needs across the various food groups.

ALL CALORIES ARE NOT CREATED EQUAL

As I've said, calories are a useful but limited concept when it comes to determining the true role of food in dictating health. For example, the same caloric amount of carrots and ice cream vary in other important attributes and thus have drastically different effects on both your health and how full they make you feel.

Let's compare a cup and a half of fruit juice against a third of a cup of almonds to help understand how and why this is. Although both contain 250 calories, they have drastically different effects on our bodies. Most juice varieties contain little to no fiber, whereas almonds are a fiber-rich food. Fiber is important for your digestive health but also helps you enjoy that full feeling that will keep hunger at bay. Juice contains little to no protein, whereas almonds are a good source of protein. Protein helps you feel satisfied, and also gives your metabolism a boost because it requires extra energy from your body to break down. Generally speaking, solid foods keep us much fuller than liquids. But don't worry—sometimes you will be in the mood for juice instead of almonds, and that's perfectly fine.

Although hunger is not the only thing that leads us to want to eat, it's obviously an important driver of food consumption. The more satiating foods you can incorporate into your diet, the better you will be able to control your hunger. Feeling full and satisfied stops hunger. As you saw with the example above and will continue to see in the chapters to come, the DASH way of eating is chock-full of nutrient-dense, fiber-rich whole foods that will keep you feeling both satisfied and nourished.

A Holistic Approach

As a dietitian, I believe strongly that the way you eat is the single greatest thing you can improve to alter the quality of your life, but I am also not naive enough to think that it's the only thing that matters. When I speak of a holistic approach to your health, what I really mean is that there are things outside of your dietary pattern that you need to keep in mind to reach your full potential.

Taking control of these other factors will put you in a better position to succeed with your dietary changes. To give you a great example of why this is, let's talk about a situation most everyone has encountered in their lives: stress eating. Sometimes, despite our best efforts and intentions, we turn to food to offer us comfort on our most challenging days. It's something that many of us, myself included, have gone through. Whether it's personal or work-related, it happens. But what happens when those stressful days start building up? If we continue to rely on food as a coping mechanism, it could seriously derail our healthy-eating and weight-management goals. That is exactly why it's so important to explore stress-management mechanisms that don't involve food.

Calling a friend, taking a walk, or even reading a book or magazine are all alternative strategies that I personally employ and that can be leveraged to avoid using food to remedy a stressful state. You might even consider seeking out a local or online stress-management training course. In fact, in a 2016 study published in the *Journal of Molecular Biochemistry*, an eight-week stress-management program led to weight loss in study participants. This type of finding provides fascinating insights into why looking beyond food is valuable and even necessary.

Let's talk about why nutrition, exercise, stress management, and sleep are critical pillars of success on your journey to better health.

NUTRITION

According to the World Health Organization, unhealthy diets and excessive energy intakes are among the primary drivers for chronic disease worldwide. Nutrition is the first and arguably most important pillar of your holistic approach to healthier living. Thus far I have spoken at great length about both the DASH diet and its ability to offer you a path to lower blood pressure as well as about the science of calories and how managing your caloric intake is an important step to take on the path toward weight loss. As you will see in the chapters to come, your 28-day DASH diet plan keeps this in mind while also offering you support for the other major pillars of health, including exercise, sleep, and stress management.

EXERCISE

As Hippocrates said, "Walking is man's best medicine." There is no question about the strong association that exists between exercise and good health. Regular physical activity is good for your heart and a key component to living a longer and healthier life. A 2012 article published in the journal *ISRN Cardiology* claimed that burning about 1,000 kcal per week through physical activity represents the threshold beyond which exercise can have a tangible positive effect on longevity. Keep in mind that you can burn this number of calories in a week simply by walking an hour a day at the pace of about three and a half miles per hour. In other words, it's important to realize you don't need to be an all-star athlete to enjoy the benefits of exercise. Further to this point, a large 2017 study published in *The Lancet* found that both recreational and nonrecreational physical activity are linked with a lower risk of heart disease.

STRESS MANAGEMENT

According to an American Psychological Association (APA) survey from 2010, 44 percent of Americans reported increased stress levels over the past five years. It's impossible to deny that stress is a pervasive component of daily life for many Americans and one that can have profound negative consequences on blood pressure, body weight, and overall health.

The authors of a 2009 study published in the *American Journal of Epidemiology* found that higher levels of stress were associated with a greater amount of weight gain over time. Above all else, stress is simply unpleasant to endure in the long term. It may be unavoidable, and it's something we all have to face from time to time, but that does not change the fact that learning how to properly manage stress is an important area of concern and one that will be discussed at greater length as part of the 28-day plan in order to help facilitate your overall success with the DASH diet.

SLEEP

There is no question that sleeping well is a very underrated cornerstone of good health. Even if everything else is going perfectly, if you are consistently sleeping too little it will probably be challenging for you to truly feel your best. Perhaps unsurprisingly, the CDC statistics suggest that one in three Americans does not reach the minimum recommendation of seven hours of sleep.

Why is this a particular problem when it comes to high blood pressure? A 2013 systematic review published in the journal *Current Pharmaceutical Design* found that insufficient sleep is linked with an increased risk of high blood pressure and hypertension. The researchers behind this particular study believe this may be due to excessive stimulation of your body's systems when too many hours are spent in a waking state, which acts as a kind of blood-pressure-raising stress, not necessarily different from other stressors one might face in daily life.

It doesn't end there, though. There is mounting evidence that sleep plays an important role in modulating your metabolism, especially as it relates to how your body responds to key hormones such as insulin, ghrelin, and leptin. According to a 2011 review in *Current Opinion in Clinical Nutrition and Metabolic Care*, a lack of sleep may also be associated with increased hunger and appetite, which may partially explain a potential relationship between sleep loss and weight gain.

Identify Counterproductive Habits

Taking strides toward healthier eating is not about turning your life upside down, but it will involve some self-reflection. Ask yourself what you are most proud of with your current eating style and what you'd like to improve upon. This type of reflection is often incredibly helpful because it encourages you to think deeply about your goals and behaviors. You are the expert on you, and the feedback that you come up with about yourself is just as valuable as the feedback that a professional can give you.

Keep in mind that this is not an exercise that stems from a place of negativity or self-criticism; rather, it's from a place of honest self-reflection. You should be proud of the positive steps you are taking to improve your health while also being aware of the behaviors that may be holding you back from your goals. The weekly habit tracker that accompanies your 28-day plan will be a very helpful tool to help facilitate this self-reflection and put you on the path to healthier habits.

But what is an unproductive habit? It is not a *bad* or *damaging* habit, but it may be an unhelpful one. Although each and every one of us lives our life in a unique way, there are certainly some common habits within this category that pop up quite often with my private practice clients.

Frequent meals out: There is nothing wrong with eating out, but when we eat out frequently we put ourselves in a position where our intake of both calories and sodium are very high, making it difficult to manage weight and lower blood pressure.

Lack of planning snacks: The large gap between lunch and dinner can be a treacherous time for many people. When hunger goes uncontrolled in this time period, it often results in either eating whatever happens to be around or being so hungry at dinnertime that less-than-ideal choices are often made.

Overusing oil: Oil offers us a healthy source of dietary fat and a way to enhance the taste of meals, but using more than 1 tablespoon of oil at a time is an easy way to overconsume calories that don't really offer you much satiety in return.

Eating out of stress or boredom: Call a friend, go for a walk, take a bath, read a book, exercise. There are a plethora of solutions at your disposal aside from food that can be used to help you avoid the common pitfall of eating to address an emotional state. Find the one that works for you, and remember there is pretty much never a bad time for a healthy snack like a piece of fruit.

Setting Goals

Success in losing weight and lowering blood pressure depends largely on your ability to effectively acclimate to the DASH style of eating. You should set goals focused on exactly that. Changes to your health and weight can come only after you've successfully embraced the wholesome, balanced style of DASH eating. Using vegetable intake as an example, let's take a look at how you can plan a SMART goal:

Specific: Be very specific. For example, I will increase my weekly vegetable intake.

Measurable: Put a number on it. For example, I will eat five servings of vegetables a day.

Achievable: Evaluate where you are relative to where you need to be. If you are eating zero servings a day right now, jumping to five may be unrealistic.

Relevant: Eating more vegetables is directly relevant to your ultimate goal of adhering to the DASH diet and plays an incredibly important role in lowering your blood pressure and keeping you full, nourished, and satisfied.

Time Bound: Setting a time frame holds you accountable to your goal. You might consider your 28-day program period as a suitable initial time frame for goal-setting purposes. Or you might want to break goals into one-week increments.

For those who may be wondering about realistic weight-loss goals, let me start by saying that I recommend thinking in the medium to long term. Thinking in months rather than days and weeks will help you enjoy healthy eating on a daily basis and remove unrealistic expectations some people place on themselves when trying to lose weight. What we know, from a health perspective, is that it takes only a modest weight loss of 5 to 10 percent of your current weight to improve indicators of metabolic functioning. In my private practice, I find my clients often realize that once they've lost around this amount of weight, they tend to report better performance in physical activity, their waist circumference decreases, their clothes start fitting better, and they ultimately don't feel the same desire to pursue further weight loss.

To put this into perspective, a 5 to 10 percent weight loss for someone who weighs 200 pounds ends up being between 10 and 20 pounds. This is no small number, but it isn't an exorbitant one either. Slow and steady advancement to that goal, which may be anywhere from four ounces to one pound a week, is a reasonable barometer of progression in those aiming to lose weight.

Please remember that the rate of loss will vary from person to person. Losing weight is hard, and your success on this program is not defined by your weight loss. Your ability to commence and maintain weight loss will hinge on a number of factors but especially finding a diet and exercise pattern within this program that you can enjoy and sustain for the long haul. For those who don't experience weight loss at the rate they anticipated, please don't lose sight of the fact that in the original DASH diet studies, participants lowered their blood pressure and improved their health *without changes to their body weight*. No matter your goal, the DASH diet will lead to a healthier you.

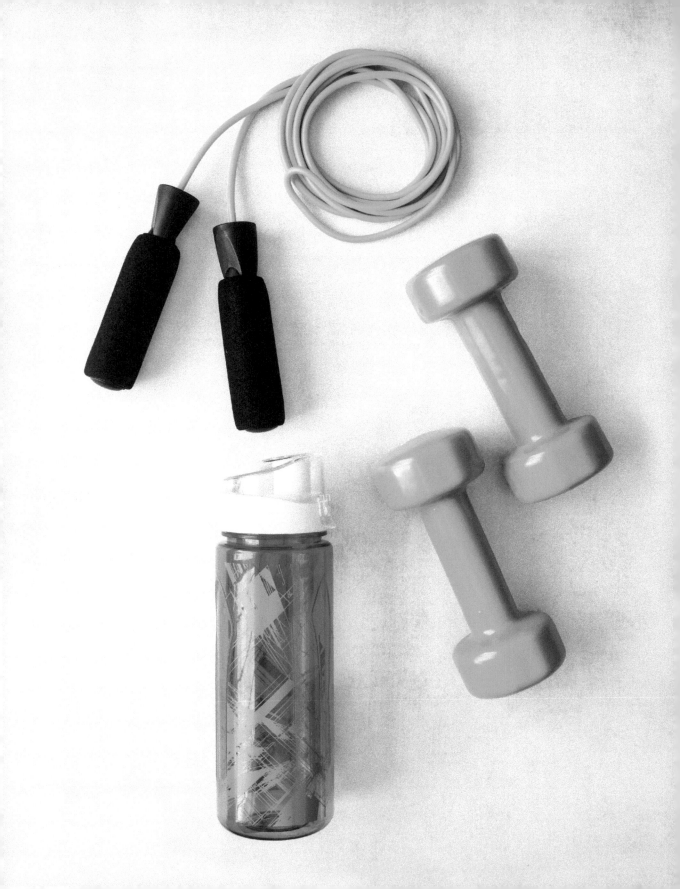

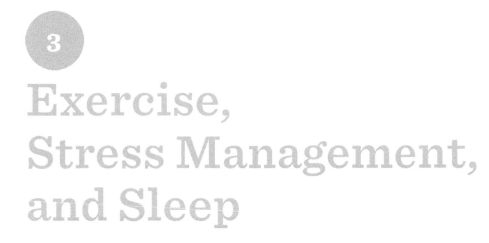

Exercise,
Stress Management,
and Sleep

Following the DASH style of eating is obviously a massive component of your 28-day plan, but it's not the only key to your success. This chapter will teach you about the additional steps you can to take to grasp control of the three other critical pillars of good health: exercise, stress management, and sleep. My clients who get the most benefit from their dietary changes are the ones who take control over other aspects of their lifestyle. It should come as no surprise that better stress management, a longer night's sleep, and regular exercise can be serious factors when it comes to losing weight.

Exercise Regularly

Exercise is good for human health in many ways, regardless of what you choose to do. My goal in this section is not only to gently introduce you to the numerous health benefits that regular physical activity can offer but also to remind you that your 28-day plan will include a diverse, varied exercise routine that I hope provides options that everyone can get something out of.

Although the DASH diet focuses on food choices, there is no denying that regular and varied exercise represents an important component of a healthy lifestyle and one that can confer additional benefits. For those of you who are starting from square one, you should know that any exercise is better than none and that there is absolutely nothing wrong with starting slowly and easing into a more rigorous routine. With that being said, the CDC identifies moderate intensity aerobic activity that totals 120 to 150 minutes weekly, in combination with two additional weekly days of muscular resistance training, as an ideal combination to confer numerous health benefits to adults. Per the CDC, these benefits include the following:

Better weight management: When combined with dietary modification, regular physical activity plays a role in supporting or enhancing weight-management efforts. Regular exercise is a great way to expend calories on top of any dietary changes you will be making on this program.

Reduced risk for cardiovascular disease: A reduction in blood pressure is a well-recognized benefit of regular physical activity, which ultimately contributes to a reduced risk of cardiovascular disease.

Reduced risk of type 2 diabetes: Regular physical activity is known to improve blood glucose control and insulin sensitivity.

Improved mood: Regular physical activity is associated with improvements in mood and reductions in anxiety owing to the manner in which exercise positively influences the biochemistry of the human brain by releasing hormones and affecting neurotransmitters.

Better sleep: Those who exercise more regularly tend to sleep better than those who don't, which may be partially owing to the reductions in stress and anxiety that often occur in those who exercise regularly.

Stronger bones and muscles: Combining cardiovascular and resistance training confers serious benefits to both your bones and your muscles, which keep your body functioning at a high level as you age.

A longer life span: Those who exercise regularly tend to enjoy a lower risk of chronic disease and a longer life span.

As you will see in the 28-day plan, your recommended exercise totals will be met by exercising four out of the seven days a week. The exercise days will be broken up as follows: All four of the active days will include aerobic exercise for 30 minutes. As a beginner, I encourage you to start slowly and build up to the four days. Two of the four active days will also include strength training. The bottom line is that you don't have to exercise for hours each day to enjoy the health benefits of physical activity. Our goal with this plan is to make the health benefits of exercise as accessible and attainable as possible for those who are ready and willing to give it a try. Before we get to the good stuff, though, there is still a lot of wisdom to be shared about getting the most out of your workouts.

GETTING THE MOST OUT OF YOUR WORKOUTS

Just as with healthy eating strategies, there are certainly important things to keep in mind about physical activity that will help support your long-term success. Let's take a look at a few important considerations that will help you get the most out of your workouts:

Rest days: Even though we haven't even started, I'm going to preach the importance of good rest. Don't forget that you are taking part in this journey to improve your health for the long term, not to burn yourself out in 28 days. Although some of you with more experience with exercise may feel confident going above and beyond, my best advice for the majority of those reading is to listen to your body and take days off to minimize risk of injury and burnout.

Stretching: Stretching is a great way to prevent injury and keep you pain-free both during workouts and in daily life. Whether it's a deliberate activity after a workout or through additional means such as yoga, stretching is beneficial in many ways.

Enjoyment: There is no right or wrong style of exercise. You are being provided a diverse plan that emphasizes a variety of different cardiovascular and resistance training exercises. If there are certain activities within these groups that you don't enjoy, it's okay not to do them. Your ability to stick with regular physical activity in the long term will depend on finding a style of exercise that you enjoy.

Your limits: Physical activity is good for you, and it should be fun, too. It's up to you to keep it that way. While it is important to challenge yourself, don't risk injury by taking things too far too fast.

Your progress: Although this is not an absolute requirement, some of you reading may find joy and fulfillment through tracking your exercise progress and striving toward a longer duration, more repetitions, and so on. If you are the type who enjoys a competitive edge, it may be fun to find a buddy to exercise and progress with.

Warm-ups: Last but certainly not least, your exercise routine will benefit greatly from a proper warm-up routine, which includes starting slowly or doing exercises similar to the ones included in your workout, but at a lower intensity.

SET A ROUTINE

The exercise part of the DASH plan was developed with CDC exercise recommendations in mind in order to support your best health. For some, the 28-day plan may seem like a lot; for others it may not seem like that much. If we look at any exercise routine from a very general perspective, there are at least three broad categories to be aware of.

Strength training: This involves utilizing your muscles against some form of counterweight, which may be your own body or dumbbells. These types of activities alter your resting metabolic rate by supporting the development of muscle while also strengthening your bones.

Aerobic exercise: Also known as cardiovascular activity, these are the quintessential exercises such as jogging or running that involve getting your body moving and getting your heart rate up.

Mobility, flexibility, and balance: Stretching after workouts or even devoting your exercise time on one day a week to stretching or yoga is a great way to maintain mobility and prevent injury in the long term.

This routine recommends involving a combination of both cardiovascular and resistance training. You will be provided with a wide array of options to choose from to accommodate a diverse exercise routine. My best recommendation is to settle on the types of exercises that offer a balance between enjoyment and challenge. Remember that the benefits of physical activity are to be enjoyed well beyond just your 28-day plan, and the best way to ensure that is the case is selecting movements you truly enjoy. My final recommendation in this regard is to also include some form of stretching either after your workouts or on a rest day.

Cardio and Body Weight Exercises

Your 28-day plan will be built around the cardiovascular and strength-training exercises that are detailed in this section. In addition to a variety of different cardiovascular exercise options, the strength-training options you will be provided are divided into four distinct categories: core, lower body, upper body, and full body. Per your sample routine, an ideal strength workout will include one exercise from each of these categories:

CARDIO

Brisk walking: This is essentially walking at a pace beyond your normal walking rate for a purpose beyond just getting from point A to point B.

Jogging: This is the intermediary stage between brisk walking and running and can be used as an accompaniment to either exercise, depending on your fitness level.

Running: The quintessential and perhaps most well-recognized cardiovascular exercise.

Jumping jacks: Although 30 minutes straight of jumping jacks may be impractical, they are a good complement to the other activities on this list.

Dancing: Those who have a background in dancing may enjoy using it to their advantage, but anyone can put on their favorite songs and dance like there's nobody watching.

Jump rope: Own a jump rope? Why not use it as part of your cardiovascular workout? It is a fun way to get your cardio in.

Other options (equipment permitting): Activities like rowing, swimming and water aerobics, biking, and using elliptical and stair climbing machines can be great ways to exercise.

In order to meet the CDC guidelines, your goal will be to work up to a total of 30 minutes of cardiovascular activity per workout session. You may use a combination of the exercises listed. I suggest that beginners should start with brisk walking or jogging—whatever activity you are most comfortable with.

CORE

Plank: The plank is a classic core exercise that focuses on stability and strength of the muscles in the abdominal and surrounding areas. Engage your buttocks, press your forearms into the ground, and hold for 60 seconds. Beginners may start with a 15- to 30-second hold and work their way up.

Side plank: Another core classic and a plank variation that focuses more on the oblique muscles on either side of your central abdominals. Keep the buttocks tight, and prevent your torso from sagging to get the most out of this exercise.

Wood chopper: A slightly more dynamic movement that works the rotational functionality of your core and mimics chopping a log of wood. You can start with little to no weight until you feel comfortable and progress from there. Start the move with feet shoulder width apart, back straight, and slightly crouched. If you are using weight, hold it with both hands next to the outside of either thigh, twist to the side, and lift the weight across and upward, keeping your arms straight and turning your torso such that you end up with the weight above your opposite shoulder.

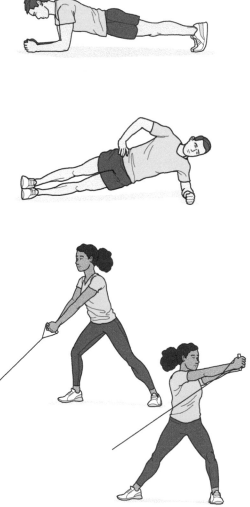

LOWER BODY

Goblet squat: Start your stance with feet slightly wider than shoulder width and a dumbbell held tightly with both hands in front of your chest. Sit back into a squat, hinging at both the knee and the hip joint, and lower your legs until they are parallel to the ground. Push up through your heels to the starting position and repeat. Use a chair to squat onto if you don't feel comfortable.

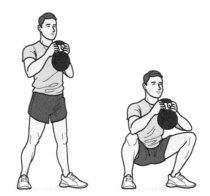

Dumbbell walking lunge: Start upright with a dumbbell in each hand and feet in your usual standing position. Step forward with one leg and sink down until your back knee is just above the ground. Remain upright and ensure the front knee does not bend over the toes. Push through the heel of the front foot and step forward and through with your rear foot. Start with no weights, and add weight as you feel comfortable.

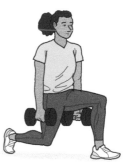

Romanian dead lift: Unlike the squat and lunge, the Romanian dead lift puts the primary emphasis on the rear muscles of the legs (hamstrings). Stand in a similar starting position to walking lunges, but this time you will hinge at the hips and push your buttocks and hip backward while naturally lowering the dumbbells in front of you. Squeeze your buttocks on the ascent back to the starting position. You can also do this exercise on one leg to improve balance and increase core activation—however, you may need to use lighter weights.

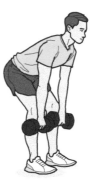

UPPER BODY

Push-ups: These are the ultimate body-weight exercise and can be done just about anywhere. You will want to set up with your hands just beyond shoulder width, keeping your body in a straight line and always engaging your core as you ascend and descend, without letting your elbows flare out. Those who struggle to perform push-ups consecutively can start by performing them on their knees or even against a wall if regular push-ups sound like too much.

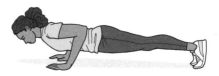

Single arm dumbbell rows: One of the more popular exercises you can do to improve the strength of your back muscles. Start with one knee and hand on an exercise bench or other flat, firm surface. Keep your back flat and your head up. Grasp the dumbbell with your free hand, with palms facing in. Reach forward and extended slightly. Bring the weight up, keeping your elbow close to your side. Hold and contract for one to two seconds, then release back to starting position.

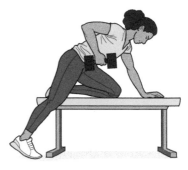

Dumbbell shoulder press: A great exercise for upper-body and shoulder strength. Bring a pair of dumbbells to ear level, palms forward, and straighten your arms overhead.

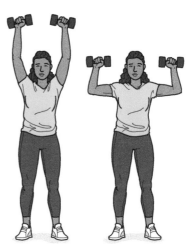

FULL BODY

Mountain climbers: On your hands and feet, keep your body in a straight line, with your abdominal and buttocks muscles engaged, similar to the top position of a push-up. Rapidly alternate pulling your knees into your chest while keeping your core tight. Continue in this left, right, left, right rhythm as if you are replicating a running motion. Always try to keep your spine in a straight line.

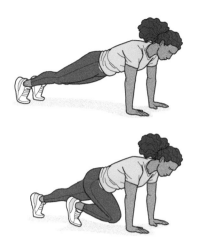

Push press: This is essentially a combination move incorporating a partial squat and a dumbbell shoulder press. Using a weight that you are comfortable with, stand feet slightly beyond shoulder width, with light dumbbells held in a pressing position. Descend for a squat to a depth you feel comfortable with, and on the ascent simultaneously push the dumbbells overhead.

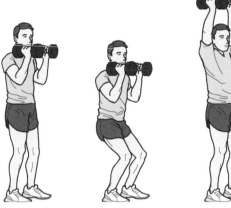

Burpee (advanced/optional):

This is a classic full-body exercise that is essentially a dynamic combination of a push-up, a squat, and a jump. This particular exercise is very effective but may be challenging for some and should be utilized only by those who feel comfortable. The proper sequencing of the movement involves starting from a standing position before lowering into a squat, placing your hands on the floor, and jumping backward to land on the balls of your feet while keeping your core strong. Jump back to your hands and jump again into the air, reaching your hands upward.

Stay Hydrated

Proper hydration by drinking water is an important habit that supports good health and weight management. Caloric drinks with minimal nutrients, like soda, have become an increasingly common source of calories in our population, and replacing such beverages with plain drinking water is a valuable step to take toward better health. Using natural flavors like a splash of lemon is a good way to transition from drinking sweetened beverages to plain water. It is recommended that women drink about 11 cups a day and men drink about 14 cups a day. Keep in mind that this includes fluid from both foods and beverages, not just water. Certain types of food, especially fruit and certain vegetables, have very high water contents. Beverages such as coffee, tea, and carbonated water also count toward your daily totals. Drinking enough water will also help prevent constipation and work together with the fiber from your diet to keep your bowels working effectively.

EXERCISE MYTHS

Myth #1: Strength training makes you bigger everywhere.

I often speak with people who refrain from strength training because they fear it will contribute to an overall bulkier appearance. Although muscular growth can certainly be a by-product of strength training, among different types of physical activity studied by the *Obesity* research journal in 2014, strength training was most strongly associated with minimizing the number of inches people added to their waists as they aged. In other words, you aren't adding size where you don't want it.

Myth #2: Weight loss always equals fat loss.

As I've alluded to throughout this book, your body weight alone can often be misleading in terms of assessing your overall health. According to a 2016 systematic review and meta-analysis published in the *Obesity Reviews* journal, loss of body weight is not the only indicator of fat loss. According to the study, although both diet and exercise can contribute to weight loss, adding exercise may be slightly more effective when it comes to specifically reducing body fat. These findings speak to the importance of the synergy between diet and exercise.

Myth #3: Aerobic exercise is all you need.

Aerobic exercise is incredibly important for your health, but according to a 2011 study published in the *American Journal of Medicine*, aerobic exercise *alone* is not very effective at encouraging weight loss or reductions in waist circumference. This is precisely why a balanced approach to resistance and cardiovascular exercise, as well as dietary changes, is important to support those with weight-loss ambitions.

Stress Management

There are undeniable connections among chronic stress, weight gain, and blood pressure. Although we can't always control how stressful our lives are, there are certainly steps that each and every one of us can take to better manage the stress we do encounter. Let's take a look at three unique strategies you can employ to help better manage your stress:

Exercise regularly: It should come as no surprise that in a book all about diet and exercise, I'm going to identify exercise as a very important stress-management strategy. Even lower-intensity workouts can make a big difference in overall health. A recent study published in the journal *Health & Place* showed that the simple act of taking a walk outdoors can help lower your stress levels.

Meditate: Meditation is a form of mindfulness that can reap immediate benefits in terms of changing the tide of a stressful day. So many of us are constantly burdened by all of the things going on in our lives, including our own expectations of ourselves and what we face ahead of us in both the short and long term. Secular mindfulness meditation, which can be done in a quiet room in a seated position with your eyes open or closed, is all about breathing naturally while focusing only on the breath and how your body responds to it. You don't want to control the breath, nor do you want your mind to wander. Start with two to three minutes daily—believe me, it's more challenging than it sounds. Need more support or an extra push? Try a meditation smartphone application such as Calm, Headspace, and The Mindfulness App.

Seek the help of friends and family: Share what's on your mind with someone who you trust but who is not directly related to what is causing you stress. We often underestimate the value of simply getting things off our chests and the effects of simple pleasures like smiling and laughter in helping us mediate the effects of a stressful day.

OVERCOMING YOUR INNER CRITIC

We've all heard the expression that you are your own harshest critic. It tends to ring true for most of us because, quite frankly, so many people find it easier to display compassion for someone else than they do for themselves. This is where mindful self-compassion comes into play. Just like it sounds, mindful self-compassion is a two-step process. Mindfulness, the first step, is the act of becoming intimately aware of what is going on in the present moment. It is a skill that can often be enhanced through various types of meditation. Why is it so important to stay in the present? Constant worrying and rumination can have detrimental effects on your mental health, which in turn may detract from your ability to successfully carry out your nutrition goals.

The second step to this process is self-compassion, which essentially means affording yourself the same understanding that you might afford a loved one who is confronting similar changes or challenges. Changing the way you eat is not easy. It's not supposed to be. No matter how close or far you are from your goals or how quickly you are able to adopt the dietary guidance provided in this book, give yourself credit for the good you've done so far. In other words, don't hesitate to act as your own cheerleader.

The ability to be compassionate toward oneself, much like the ability to be mindful and present, is conducive to better overall mental health, which in turn will support your success in pursuing the guidance that this book provides.

Sleep

According to the joint consensus statement of both the American Academy of Sleep Medicine and the Sleep Research Society, the recommended level of daily sleep for most adults is at least seven hours but no more than eight. For those who sleep below the recommended minimum of seven hours, there is a growing body of evidence linking insufficient sleep and poor health outcomes. A 2006 study published in the journal *Sleep* found that individuals who slept less than seven hours a night, and especially those who slept under six, had a higher risk of hypertension. Interestingly enough, a 2008 study from the same journal found sleep duration that was either below (five to six hours) or above (nine to ten hours) recommended levels was associated with weight gain.

If you regularly sleep under seven hours a night, or generally have trouble sleeping well, it may be time to reevaluate your sleep hygiene. For those who may not have heard of this term before, a person's sleep habits are often referred to as their sleep hygiene, and just like good oral hygiene means a good report at your next dentist visit, good sleep hygiene is conducive to a good night's sleep. The CDC recommends focusing on the following things to improve your sleep hygiene:

Consistency: Going to sleep and waking up at similar times all seven days a week.

Ambience: Ensuring the bedroom is conducive to sleep by offering a dark, quiet setting at a cool, comfortable temperature. Some of you will prefer slightly warmer or slightly cooler settings, so don't be afraid to experiment to figure out what you feel works best.

Avoid electronics: Make it a hard-and-fast rule to keep your bedroom an electronics-free zone. That includes cell phones! Consider shutting off your devices at least an hour before bedtime and relying on an alarm clock, rather than your phone alarm, to wake you up in the morning. This will make you less reliant on having your phone on or near you while you sleep.

Avoid large amounts of food and drink: Some people may find it easier to sleep if they avoid larger meals or drinking beverages like coffee or alcohol before bedtime. A soothing herbal tea may be an exception to this rule, though.

Physical activity: Being more physically active during the day, rather than later at night, may help you fall asleep more easily.

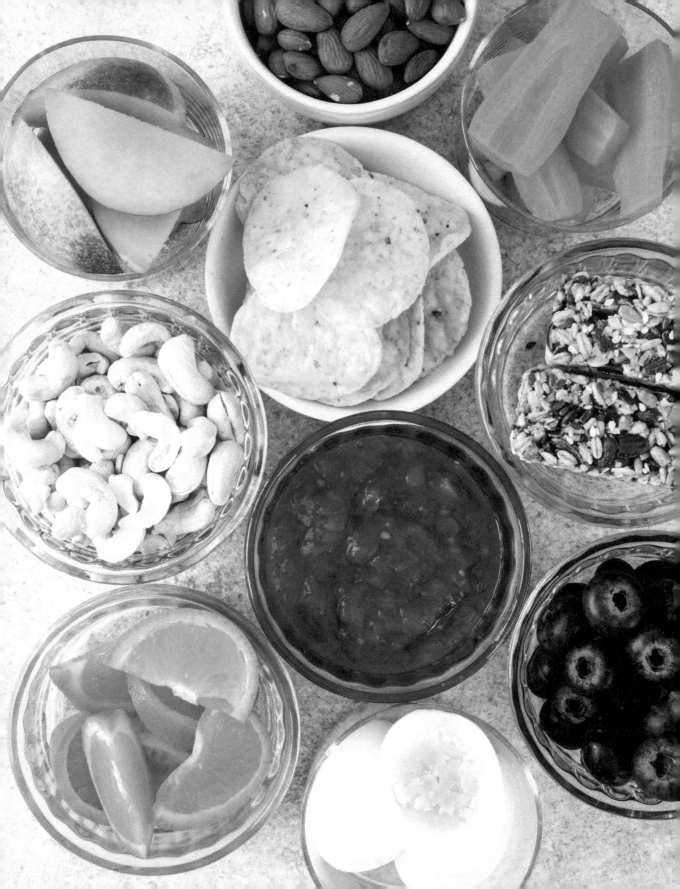

4

The 28-Day Program and Beyond

You now have all of the tools you need to assemble a healthier lifestyle, but you still don't have the blueprint for how to put the moving parts together. That's exactly what this section of the book provides. The 28-day program will lay out the exact steps you need to take, including detailed and delicious meal plans, in order to make those first major strides toward success with the DASH eating style. Let's get started! The weekly meal plans that follow are based on a 1,600 calories intake per day. Those with higher or lower calorie needs can use the calorie-specific tables to approximate and adjust their intake via increasing or decreasing their portion sizes at meals or incorporating extra snacks or side dishes, to meet their differing needs across the various food groups. One of the greatest tools this book offers you is the extensive list of recipes created by the talented Julie Andrews. Together, Julie and I developed extensive nutrition criteria for our recipes to ensure they are DASH diet-friendly. In other words, you can be confident that the recipes you have at your disposal are high in nutrients you need and low in sodium you don't.

Pantry, Refrigerator, and Freezer Staples

Planning meals and snacks for the week can become simpler, quicker, and easier when you have a few staples in your pantry, fridge, and freezer. We've compiled a list of some of the items you'll use regularly throughout the 28-day program and beyond.

Many of these items are building blocks for well-balanced meals, while other ingredients provide balance, add flavor, or give a boost of nutrition to your recipes. You should plan to have these ingredients on hand, as they are not covered in the weekly shopping lists that follow. Take a moment to go through your pantry, refrigerator, and freezer to see what items you may be missing and add them to your next shop.

Pantry Basics

- All-purpose and whole-wheat flour
- Apple cider vinegar
- Baking powder
- Baking soda
- Balsamic vinegar
- Bay leaves
- Black pepper
- Canola or avocado oil
- Celery seeds
- Chili powder
- Cooking spray
- Cornstarch
- Crushed red pepper flakes
- Dark brown sugar
- Dark chocolate chips
- Dried dill
- Dried Mexican oregano leaves
- Dried mustard powder
- Dried oregano leaves
- Dried sage
- Extra-virgin olive oil
- Garam masala (make your own, page 215)
- Garlic powder
- Granulated stevia
- Granulated sugar
- Ground cayenne pepper
- Ground cinnamon
- Ground cumin
- Ground flaxseed
- Ground ginger
- Ground nutmeg
- Honey
- Hot sauce
- Italian seasoning
- Kosher or sea salt
- Low-sodium taco seasoning (make your own, page 216)
- Old-fashioned rolled oats
- Onion powder
- Panko bread crumbs
- Pitted dates
- Pumpkin pie spice
- Pure vanilla extract
- Red wine vinegar
- Rice wine vinegar
- Sesame oil
- Sesame seeds
- Smoked paprika
- Sriracha
- Unsweetened coconut flakes
- White wine vinegar
- Whole-wheat pastry flour
- Worcestershire sauce
- Yellow cornmeal

Refrigerator and Freezer Staples

- Dijon and yellow mustard
- Lower-sodium ketchup
- Mayonnaise
- Minced onion
- Unsalted butter
- Unsalted stock, vegetable or chicken and beef (make your own and freeze, page 217)

Week 1

You have to take your first step before you can take your second.

Week 1 is all about taking your first steps to success. You shouldn't be concerned about perfection. Depending on your starting point, week 1 may represent a pretty significant divergence from your previous diet and exercise pattern. Not to be overly dramatic, but I want you to think of week 1 more like the first week of the rest of your life, as opposed to the first week of a 28-day plan. The reality remains that healthy eating and physical activity are lifelong endeavors that should be pursued with consistency and regularity in order to have the best effect on your health. With that in mind, celebrate small steps toward your goal and know that you have plenty of weeks ahead to continue to develop routine, familiarity, and comfort with the DASH diet.

WEEK 1 MEAL PLAN

Monday

Breakfast
Broccoli Cheese Egg Muffins (page 86)

1 cup or medium piece fresh fruit

Lunch
Mediterranean Chickpea Tuna Salad (page 103)

7 to 8 whole-grain crackers

Dinner
Italian-Style Turkey Meat Loaf (page 167)

Lemony Green Beans with Almonds (page 197)

Snacks
2 to 3; midmorning, midafternoon, and evening

Tuesday

Breakfast
Peach Avocado Smoothie (page 80)

1 hard-boiled or scrambled egg

Lunch
Leftover Italian-Style Turkey Meat Loaf (page 167)

Leftover Lemony Green Beans with Almonds (page 197)

Dinner
Crispy Fish Sandwiches with Creamy Coleslaw (page 120)

1 cup cooked vegetables

Snacks
2 to 3; midmorning, midafternoon, and evening

Wednesday

Breakfast
Broccoli Cheese Egg Muffins (page 86)

1 cup or medium piece fresh fruit

Lunch
Leftover Crispy Fish Sandwiches with Creamy Coleslaw (page 120)

1 cup cooked vegetables

Dinner
Grilled Pork & Pineapple Kebabs (page 179)

½ cup Fluffy Brown Rice (page 223)

Snacks
2 to 3; midmorning, midafternoon, and evening

Thursday

Breakfast
Morning Glory Smoothie (page 79)

1 hard-boiled or scrambled egg

Lunch
Leftover Grilled Pork & Pineapple Kebabs (page 179)

½ cup leftover Fluffy Brown Rice (page 223)

Dinner
Turkey Taco Weeknight Skillet (page 166)

1 cup or medium piece fresh fruit

Snacks
2 to 3; midmorning, midafternoon, and evening

Friday

Breakfast
Broccoli Cheese Egg Muffins (page 86)

1 cup or medium piece fresh fruit

Lunch
Leftover Turkey Taco Weeknight Skillet (page 166)

1 cup or medium piece fresh fruit

Dinner
Tofu & Green Bean Stir-Fry (page 125) with Fluffy Brown Rice (page 223)

Snacks
2 to 3; midmorning, midafternoon, and evening

Saturday

Breakfast
Roasted Red Pepper & Pesto Omelet (page 88)

1 cup or medium piece fresh fruit

Lunch
Leftover Tofu & Green Bean Stir-Fry (page 125) with Fluffy Brown Rice (page 223)

Dinner
Eggplant Parmesan Stacks (page 134)

Rustic Tomato Panzanella Salad (page 104)

Dessert
Oatmeal Dark Chocolate Chip Peanut Butter Cookie (page 203)

Snacks
1 to 2; midmorning and midafternoon

Sunday

Breakfast
Sweet Potato Pancakes with Maple Yogurt (page 92)

1 cup or medium piece fresh fruit

Lunch
Waldorf Chicken Salad (page 102) with Honey Whole-Wheat Bread (page 224)

½ cup raw vegetables

Dinner
Black Bean Stew with Cornbread (page 146)

Green salad with 2 table- spoons dressing

Dessert
Oatmeal Dark Chocolate Chip Peanut Butter Cookie (page 203)

Snacks
1 to 2; midmorning and midafternoon

Suggested Snacks
Coconut Date Energy Bite (page 191)

Sweet & Salty Nut Mix (page 195)

Medium piece fruit with 1 tablespoon natural peanut butter

6-ounce nonfat fruit-flavored Greek yogurt with ½ cup fresh fruit

1 cup bell pepper slices with 2 tablespoons hummus

WEEK 1 PREP LIST

- Chop fruit and vegetables for meals, snacks, and side dishes.
- Make Broccoli Cheese Egg Muffins (page 86).
- Prep Mediterranean Chickpea Tuna Salad (page 103).
- Make Fluffy Brown Rice (page 223).
- Prep Stir-Fry Sauce (page 222).
- Make Honey Whole-Wheat Bread (page 224), if desired, for Waldorf Chicken Salad (page 102).
- Make Coconut Date Energy Bites (page 191) and/or Sweet & Salty Nut Mix (page 195), if using for snacks.

WEEK 1 SHOPPING LIST

Produce

Apple (1)

Avocados (3)

Bananas (2)

Basil (1 container)

Broccoli (1 small head)

Carrots (3)

Celery (1 small bag)

Cilantro, fresh (1 bunch)

Coleslaw mix, 1 (10-ounce) bag

Cucumber, English (1)

Eggplant (1 large)

Fruit, fresh (8 pieces or 8 chopped cups)

Garlic (1 head)

Ginger (1 piece)

Green beans (2 pounds)

Grapes, green or red (1 small bag)

Lemons (3)

Lettuce (1 small bag shredded or 1 small head)

Limes (2)

Parsley, Italian, flat leaf, fresh (1 bunch)

Peppers, bell, red (2)

Pepper, jalapeño (1)

Pineapple (1 small)

Red onions (2)

Scallions (2)

Spinach, baby (4 cups)

Sweet potatoes (2)

Tomatoes (4–5)

Tomatoes, cherry (1 pint)

Vegetables, raw (baby carrots, cucumber, bell pepper, and others) (4 cups)

Yellow onions (2)

Dairy

Buttermilk, low fat (1 small carton)

Cheese, Cheddar, shredded (1 cup)

Cheese, feta (¼ cup)

Cheese, mozzarella, shredded (½ cup)

Cheese, mozzarella, fresh (½ pound)

Cheese, Parmesan, grated (¾ cup)

Cheese, white Cheddar, shredded (¾ cup)

Eggs, large (26)

Milk, skim (½ gallon)

Tofu, extra firm, 1 (14-ounce) package

Yogurt, nonfat fruit-flavored Greek (2 [6-ounce] containers)

Yogurt, nonfat plain Greek (1 [32-ounce] tub)

Meat, Poultry, and Fish

Chicken breast (1½ pounds)

Fish, white (cod, haddock, or tilapia) (2 pounds)

Pork tenderloin (2 pounds)

Tuna, albacore (1 [6.4-ounce] pouch)

Turkey, ground (3 pounds)

Canned, Bottled, and Dried Goods

Beans, black, no salt added (3 [15-ounce] cans)

Chickpeas, no salt added (2 [15-ounce] cans)

Crackers, whole grain (1 small box)

Juice, apple (1 small bottle)

Marinara (1 [24-ounce] jar)

Olives, kalamata (1 small jar)

Purée, sweet potato or pumpkin (1 [15-ounce] can)

Red peppers, roasted (1 small jar)

Salad dressing (1 small bottle)

Soy sauce, low sodium (1 small bottle)

Tomatoes, diced, no salt added, fire roasted (1 [10-ounce] can)

Frozen

Peaches (1½ cups)

Vegetables, cooked, any variety (2 bags)

Grains

Baguette (1 small)

Buns, sandwich, whole wheat (8)

Rice, brown (1 large bag)

Pantry Items

Almonds, sliced (¼ cup)

Almonds, whole (½ cup)

Cashews (¼ cup)

Chocolate chips, dark (1 small bag)

Coconut flakes, unsweetened (2 tablespoons)

Peanut butter, natural (1 small jar)

Pine nuts (¼ cup)

Syrup, maple, pure (1 small bottle)

Tahini (1 small jar)

Tortilla chips, whole-grain corn (1 small bag)

Walnuts, chopped (¾ cup)

YOUR EXERCISE ROUTINE

Cardio workouts should be 30 minutes in duration, but you can work up to this length if you are a beginner. Strength workouts should include 3 to 4 sets of 8 to 10 repetitions of each exercise where applicable. In the case of static core exercises such as the plank, work toward holding the movements for longer each week.

My Exercise Routine

The following is your exercise plan for the week. Fill in the table with the cardio and strength-training exercises (pages 33–37) you plan to do.

M	T	W	TH	F	SAT	S
Cardio:	**Cardio:**	R E S T	**Cardio:**	R E S T	**Cardio:**	R E S T
	Core		Core			
	Lower Body		Lower Body			
	Upper Body		Upper Body			
	Full Body		Full Body			

YOUR HABIT TRACKER

The habit tracker is an optional but very useful tool to help you keep tabs on some of the important health behaviors that are encouraged throughout the book.

Sleeping eight hours a night, meditation, and eating your recommended daily servings of vegetables are all very important habits that you could potentially choose to track using this helpful tool.

My Habit Tracker

It's important to make healthy lifestyle choices in addition to dietary changes. Create a list of healthy habits you want to maintain over the next four weeks and mark the days when you succeed.

HABIT	M	T	W	TH	F	SAT	S
Drank 8 glasses of water	X		X	X		X	

Week 2

Momentum is the strength or force that something has when it is moving.

No matter how week 1 went, the fact you've arrived on this page of the book means that you are ready for week 2. As far as I'm concerned, that means a job well done. Before we go any further, though, I want you to go through the exercise of identifying all of the things you did well this past week. Be proud of those steps. Next, I want you to identify a few of the things you know you can improve upon, and make those the focal points of week 2 as you slowly work toward your best version of the DASH diet and a healthier, more active lifestyle.

WEEK 2 MEAL PLAN

Monday

Breakfast
Roasted Root Vegetable Hash (page 90) with Perfectly Poached Eggs (page 210)

1 cup or medium piece fresh fruit

Lunch
Leftover Black Bean Stew with Cornbread (page 146)

Green salad with 2 table-spoons dressing

Dinner
Spaghetti & Chicken Meatballs (page 159)

1 cup cooked vegetables

Snacks
2 to 3; midmorning, midafter-noon, and evening

Tuesday

Breakfast
Blueberry Date Muffin (page 84)

1 hard-boiled or scrambled egg

Lunch
Leftover Spaghetti & Chicken Meatballs (page 159)

1 cup cooked vegetables

Dinner
Sweet Potato Cakes with Classic Guacamole (page 130)

1 cup or medium piece fresh fruit

Snacks
2 to 3; midmorning, midafter-noon, and evening

Wednesday

Breakfast
Roasted Root Vegetable Hash (page 90) with Perfectly Poached Eggs (page 210)

1 cup or medium piece fresh fruit

Lunch
Leftover Sweet Potato Cakes with Classic Guacamole (page 130)

1 cup or medium piece fresh fruit

Dinner
Grilled Flank Steak with Peach Compote (page 174)

Green salad with 2 table-spoons dressing

Snacks
2 to 3; midmorning, midafter-noon, and evening

Thursday

Breakfast
Blueberry Date Muffin
(page 84)
1 hard-boiled or scrambled egg

Lunch
Leftover Grilled Flank Steak
with Peach Compote
(page 174)
Green salad with 2 table-
spoons dressing

Dinner
Spicy Tofu Burrito Bowl with
Cilantro Avocado Sauce
(page 128)
1 cup or medium piece
fresh fruit

Snacks
2 to 3; midmorning, midafternoon, and evening

Friday

Breakfast
Roasted Root Vegetable
Hash (page 90) with Perfectly
Poached Eggs (page 210)
1 cup or medium piece
fresh fruit

Lunch
Leftover Spicy Tofu Burrito
Bowl with Cilantro Avocado
Sauce (page 128)
1 cup or medium piece
fresh fruit

Dinner
Chili Lime Chicken Fajitas with
Mango Salsa (page 160)

Snacks
2 to 3; midmorning, midafternoon, and evening

Saturday

Breakfast
Peanut Butter & Banana
Oatmeal (page 82)
1 cup or medium piece
fresh fruit

Lunch
Leftover Chili Lime Chicken
Fajitas with Mango Salsa
(page 160)

Dinner
Pork Tenderloin with
Balsamic Cherry Pan
Sauce (page 184)
Maple Mustard Brussels
Sprouts with Toasted Walnuts
(page 198)

Dessert
Key Lime Cherry "Nice" Cream
(page 202)

Snacks
1 to 2; midmorning and
midafternoon

Sunday

Breakfast
Greek Breakfast Scramble
(page 87)

1 slice whole-wheat toast
with 1 teaspoon
unsalted butter

Lunch
Leftover Pork Tenderloin with
Balsamic Cherry Pan Sauce
(page 184)
Leftover Maple Mustard
Brussels Sprouts with Toasted
Walnuts (page 198)

Dinner
Shrimp & Corn Chowder
(page 114)
Green salad with 2 table-
spoons dressing

Dessert
Key Lime Cherry "Nice" Cream
(page 202)

Snacks
1 to 2; midmorning and
midafternoon

Suggested Snacks
Roasted Root Vegetable Chips
with French Onion Yogurt Dip
(page 192)
Peanut Butter Banana Bread
Bite (page 206)
15 whole-grain corn tortilla
chips with ½ cup Simple
Tomato Salsa (page 211)
(leftover from week 1)
1 part-skim string cheese with
1 medium piece fruit

WEEK 2 PREP LIST

- Chop fruit and vegetables
  for meals, snacks, and
  side dishes.

- Make Roasted Root
  Vegetable Hash (page 90)
  with Perfectly Poached
  Eggs (page 210).

- Make Blueberry Date
  Muffins (page 84).

- Marinate chicken for Chili Lime Chicken Fajitas with Mango Salsa (page 160).
- Make Roasted Root Vegetable Chips and French

Onion Yogurt Dip (page 192) and Peanut Butter Banana Bread Bites (page 206), if using for snacks.

- Make Honey Whole-Wheat Bread (page 224) for toast (optional).

WEEK 2 SHOPPING LIST

Produce

Avocados (4)

Bananas (8)

Beet (1)

Brussels sprouts (2 pounds)

Carrots (2)

Cilantro (1 bunch)

Fruit, fresh (8 pieces or 8 chopped cups)

Garlic (1 head)

Kale (1 bunch or 2 cups chopped)

Limes (5)

Mango (1)

Onions, red (3)

Onions, yellow (2)

Parsley, Italian, flat leaf (1 bunch)

Parsnips (2)

Peaches (2)

Pepper, jalapeño (1)

Peppers, bell (3)

Potatoes, Yukon Gold or red (5 baby)

Scallions (2)

Spinach, baby (4 cups)

Sweet potatoes (5 small to medium)

Tomatoes, cherry (1 pint)

Vegetables, raw (baby carrots, cucumber, bell pepper, and others) (4 cups)

Dairy

Cheese, feta (1 small container)

Cheese, Parmesan, grated (2 tablespoons)

Cheese, string, part-skim (1 bag)

Eggs, large (21)

Milk, skim (½ gallon)

Tofu, extra firm (1 [14-ounce] container)

Yogurt, nonfat plain Greek (1 [32-ounce] tub)

Meat, Poultry, and Fish

Chicken breast, boneless, skinless (1 pound)

Chicken, ground (2 pounds)

Pork tenderloin (2 pounds)

Shrimp, raw, peeled and deveined (1 pound)

Steak, flank (1½ pounds)

Canned Goods

Black beans, no salt added (2 [15-ounce] cans)

Frozen

Blueberries (1 cup)

Cherries, dark, sweet (1 [12-ounce] bag)

Corn, sweet (4 cups)

Grains

Bread, whole wheat (if using for toast) (1 loaf)

Spaghetti, whole grain (1 pound)

Tortillas, corn (1 small bag)

Pantry Items

Walnuts, chopped (¼ cup)

YOUR EXERCISE ROUTINE

Cardio workouts should be 30 minutes in duration, but you can work up to this length if you are a beginner. Strength workouts should include 3 to 4 sets of 8 to 10 repetitions of each exercise where applicable. In the case of static core exercises such as the plank, work toward holding the movements for longer each week.

My Exercise Routine

The following is your exercise plan for the week. Fill in the table with the cardio and strength-training exercises (pages 33–37) you plan to do.

M	T	W	TH	F	SAT	S
Cardio:	Cardio:	R E S T	Cardio:	R E S T	Cardio:	R E S T
	Core		Core			
	Lower Body		Lower Body			
	Upper Body		Upper Body			
	Full Body		Full Body			

YOUR HABIT TRACKER

The habit tracker is an optional but very useful tool to help you keep tabs on some of the important health behaviors that are encouraged throughout the book. Sleeping eight hours a night, meditation, and eating your recommended daily servings of vegetables are all very important habits that you could potentially choose to track using this helpful tool.

My Habit Tracker

It's important to make healthy lifestyle choices in addition to dietary changes. Create a list of healthy habits you want to maintain over the next four weeks and mark the days when you succeed.

HABIT	M	T	W	TH	F	SAT	S
Drank 8 glasses of water	X		X	X		X	

Week 3

The third time is a charm.

Or, in this case, the third week is a charm. By this point my hope is that, with two solid weeks under your belt, your self-confidence and self-efficacy are both growing, and the completion of this third week will be a tipping point for continued progress in the last week of the 28-day plan and beyond. Ideally, I'd love you to feel like the DASH diet has become more of a natural process. Now is the time to be honest with yourself about any part of the eating plan that may not be working for you. It will be up to you to use week 3 to try alternative approaches, foods, or exercises to help address those concerns so that they don't linger and become problematic further down the line.

WEEK 3 MEAL PLAN

Monday

Breakfast
Mushroom Thyme Frittata (page 89)

1 cup or medium piece fresh fruit

Lunch
Avocado Egg Salad (page 105)

½ cup raw vegetables

Dinner
Grilled Salmon with Chimichurri (page 150)

Grilled Corn & Edamame Succotash (page 196)

Snacks
2 to 3; midmorning, midafternoon, and evening

Tuesday

Breakfast
Mango Pineapple Green Smoothie (page 78)

1 hard-boiled or scrambled egg

Lunch
Avocado Egg Salad (page 105)

½ cup raw vegetables

Dinner
Roasted Vegetable Enchiladas (page 136)

Leftover Grilled Corn & Edamame Succotash (page 196)

Snacks
2 to 3; midmorning, midafternoon, and evening

Wednesday

Breakfast
Mushroom Thyme Frittata (page 89)

1 cup or medium piece fresh fruit

Lunch
Leftover Roasted Vegetable Enchiladas (page 136)

1 cup or medium piece fresh fruit

Dinner
Chickpea Cauliflower Tikka Masala (page 132)

Green salad with 2 tablespoons dressing

Snacks
2 to 3; midmorning, midafternoon, and evening

Thursday

Breakfast

Mango Pineapple Green Smoothie (page 78)

1 hard-boiled or scrambled egg

Lunch

Leftover Chickpea Cauliflower Tikka Masala (page 132)

Green salad with 2 tablespoons dressing

Dinner

Turkey & Rice–Stuffed Cabbage Rolls (page 168)

1 cup or medium piece fresh fruit

Snacks

2 to 3; midmorning, midafternoon, and evening

Friday

Breakfast

Mushroom Thyme Frittata (page 89)

1 cup or medium piece fresh fruit

Lunch

Leftover Turkey & Rice–Stuffed Cabbage Rolls (page 168)

Green salad with 2 tablespoons dressing

Dinner

Slow Cooker Beef Ragu with Creamy Polenta (page 180)

1 cup cooked vegetables

Snacks

2 to 3; midmorning, midafternoon, and evening

Saturday

Breakfast

Whole-Grain Flax Waffles with Strawberry Purée (page 94)

1 cup or medium piece fresh fruit

Lunch

Leftover Slow Cooker Beef Ragu with Creamy Polenta (page 180)

1 cup cooked vegetables

Dinner

Indian-Spiced Chicken Kebabs (page 158)

Fennel & Grape Potato Salad with Tarragon Dressing (page 200)

Dessert

Grilled Plums with Vanilla Bean Frozen Yogurt (page 201)

Snacks

1 to 2; midmorning and midafternoon

Sunday

Breakfast

Sweet Potato Pancakes with Maple Yogurt (page 92)

1 cup or medium piece fresh fruit

Lunch

Leftover Indian-Spiced Chicken Kebabs (page 158)

Leftover Fennel & Grape Potato Salad with Tarragon Dressing (page 200)

Dinner

Classic Beef & Bean Chili (page 116)

Green salad with 2 tablespoons dressing

Dessert

Grilled Plums with Vanilla Bean Frozen Yogurt (page 201)

Snacks

1 to 2; midmorning and midafternoon

Suggested Snacks

Crispy Cinnamon Apple Chips (page 190)

Stovetop Cheese Popcorn (page 194)

Medium piece fruit with 2 tablespoons natural peanut butter

6-ounce nonfat fruit-flavored Greek yogurt with ½ cup fresh fruit

1 cup bell pepper slices with 2 tablespoons yogurt ranch

WEEK 3 PREP LIST

- Chop fruit and vegetables for meals, snacks, and side dishes.
- Make Mushroom Thyme Frittata (page 89).
- Make 11 hard-boiled eggs.
- Make Avocado Egg Salad (page 105).
- Grill sweet corn for Grilled Corn & Edamame Succotash (page 196) and Roasted Vegetable Enchiladas (page 136).
- Make Fluffy Brown Rice (page 223).
- Make Crispy Cinnamon Apple Chips (page 190) and Stovetop Cheese Popcorn (page 194), if using for snacks.

WEEK 3 SHOPPING LIST

Produce

Apples (3)

Avocados (2)

Basil (1 container)

Cabbage (1 head)

Cauliflower (1 head)

Cilantro (1 bunch)

Corn, sweet (6 ears)

Eggplant (1)

Fennel (1 head)

Fruit, fresh (8 pieces or 8 chopped cups)

Garlic (1 head)

Ginger (1 piece)

Grapes, red (2 cups)

Lemons (2)

Limes (2)

Mushrooms, sliced (2 cups)

Onion, red (1)

Onions, yellow (4)

Parsley, Italian, flat leaf (1 bunch)

Pepper, jalapeño (1)

Peppers, bell (2)

Plums (4 large)

Potatoes, Yukon Gold or red (4)

Scallions (2)

Shallot (1 large)

Spinach, baby, or kale, chopped (6 to 8 cups)

Strawberries (1 quart)

Tarragon (1 container)

Thyme (1 container)

Tomatoes, cheery (2 pints)

Vegetables, raw (baby carrots, cucumber, bell pepper, and others) (4 cups)

Yogurt ranch (1 small bottle)

Zucchini (2)

Dairy

Cheese, Mexican-style, shredded (1½ cups)

Cheese, Parmesan, grated (¼ cup)

Cheese, Swiss, shredded (1½ cups)

Eggs, large (36)

Juice, orange (1¼ cups)

Milk, skim (½ gallon)

Yogurt, nonfat fruit-flavored Greek (2 [6-ounce] containers)

Yogurt, nonfat plain Greek (2 [32-ounce] tubs)

Meat, Poultry & Fish

Beef, chuck roast (2 pounds)

Chicken breast, boneless, skinless (1 pound)

Salmon (1 pound)

Turkey, ground (1½ pounds)

Canned and Bottled Goods

Beans, black, no salt added (1 [15-ounce] can)

Chickpeas or garbanzo beans, no salt added (2 [15-ounce] cans)

Milk, coconut (1 [15-ounce] can)

Purée, sweet potato or pumpkin (1 [15-ounce] can)

Salad dressing (1 small bottle)

Tomatoes, crushed, no salt added (3 [32-ounce] cans)

Tomatoes, diced, petite, no salt added (1 [15-ounce] can)

Frozen

Edamame, shelled (2 cups)

Mango, cubed (2 cups)

Pineapple, cubed (2 cups)

Yogurt, frozen, vanilla bean (1 small carton)

Grains

Popcorn, kernels (1 small bag)

Tortillas, whole wheat, 8 inch (8)

Pantry Items

Almonds, sliced (¼ cup)

Nutritional yeast flakes (1 small bottle)

YOUR EXERCISE ROUTINE

Cardio workouts should be 30 minutes in duration, but you can work up to this length if you are a beginner. Strength workouts should include 3 to 4 sets of 8 to 10 repetitions of each exercise where applicable. In the case of static core exercises such as the plank, work toward holding the movements for longer each week.

My Exercise Routine

The following is your exercise plan for the week. Fill in the table with the cardio and strength-training exercises (pages 33–37) you plan to do.

M	T	W	TH	F	SAT	S
Cardio:	**Cardio:**		**Cardio:**		**Cardio:**	
	Core		Core			
	Lower Body	R E S T	Lower Body	R E S T		R E S T
	Upper Body		Upper Body			
	Full Body		Full Body			

YOUR HABIT TRACKER

The habit tracker is an optional but very useful tool to help you keep tabs on some of the important health behaviors that are encouraged throughout the book. Sleeping eight hours a night, meditation, and eating your recommended daily servings of vegetables are all very important habits that you could potentially choose to track using this helpful tool.

My Habit Tracker

It's important to make healthy lifestyle choices in addition to dietary changes. Create a list of healthy habits you want to maintain over the next four weeks and mark the days when you succeed.

HABIT	M	T	W	TH	F	SAT	S
Drank 8 glasses of water	X		X	X		X	

Week 4

Writing the first chapter is the first step to completing a book.

Indulge me for a moment and picture your healthy eating journey as a book. You are on the verge of completing the first chapter. Yes, you have a long way to go to finish your story, but afford yourself a moment of congratulations for the commitment you've demonstrated so far. The last week of this plan represents both the end of your 28-day plan and the start of the rest of your life as a healthy, balanced, and varied eater. It's not about perfection; it's about persistence. At this point, you've learned a great deal about both yourself and the DASH diet, and you will always have this book as a resource to support you on your path toward continued success, health, and wellness. Congratulations!

WEEK 4 MEAL PLAN

Monday

Breakfast
Hash Brown Vegetable Breakfast Casserole (page 91)

1 cup or medium piece fresh fruit

Lunch
Classic Beef & Bean Chili (page 116)

Green salad with 2 table-spoons dressing

Dinner
Chicken & Mandarin Orange Salad with Sesame Ginger Dressing (page 98)

Snacks
2 to 3; midmorning, midafternoon, and evening

Tuesday

Breakfast
Hash Brown Vegetable Breakfast Casserole (page 91)

1 cup or medium piece fresh fruit

Lunch
Leftover Chicken & Mandarin Orange Salad with Sesame Ginger Dressing (page 98)

Dinner
Tomato & Olive Orecchiette with Basil Pesto (page 139)

1 cup or medium piece fresh fruit

Snacks
2 to 3; midmorning, midafternoon, and evening

Wednesday

Breakfast
Hash Brown Vegetable Breakfast Casserole (page 91)

1 cup or medium piece fresh fruit

Lunch
Leftover Tomato & Olive Orecchiette with Basil Pesto (page 139)

1 cup or medium piece fresh fruit

Dinner
Spinach & Feta Salmon Burgers (page 152)

Green salad with 2 table-spoons dressing

Snacks
2 to 3; midmorning, midafternoon, and evening

Breakfast

Apple Cinnamon Overnight Oats (page 81)

1 hard-boiled or scrambled egg

Lunch

Leftover Spinach & Feta Salmon Burgers (page 152)

Green salad with 2 tablespoons dressing

Dinner

Chicken Tortilla Casserole (page 162)

1 cup or medium piece fresh fruit

Snacks

2 to 3; midmorning, midafternoon, and evening

Breakfast

Dark Chocolate Walnut Bar (page 83)

1 cup or medium piece fresh fruit

Lunch

Leftover Chicken Tortilla Casserole (page 162)

1 cup or medium piece fresh fruit

Dinner

Salmon & Avocado Cobb Salad with Buttermilk Ranch Dressing (page 100)

Cauliflower Leek Soup (page 110)

Snacks

2 to 3; midmorning, midafternoon, and evening

Breakfast

Whole-Grain Flax Waffles with Strawberry Purée (page 94)

1 cup or medium piece fresh fruit

Lunch

Leftover Salmon & Avocado Cobb Salad with Buttermilk Ranch Dressing (page 100)

Cauliflower Leek Soup (page 110)

Dinner

Barbecue Pork Sliders with Avocado Slaw (page 186)

1 cup cooked vegetables

Dessert

Peach Crumble Muffin (page 204)

Snacks

1 to 2; midmorning and midafternoon

Breakfast

Greek Breakfast Scramble (page 87)

1 cup or medium piece fresh fruit

Lunch

Leftover Barbecue Pork Sliders with Avocado Slaw (page 186)

1 cup cooked vegetables

Dinner

Crispy Balsamic Chicken Thighs (page 153)

Caramelized Sweet Potato Wedges (page 199)

Green salad with 2 tablespoons dressing

Dessert

Peach Crumble Muffin (page 204)

Snacks

1 to 2; midmorning and midafternoon

Suggested Snacks

Dark Chocolate Walnut Bar (page 83)

Coconut Date Energy Bite (page 191)

1 part-skim string cheese with 1 medium piece fruit

1 cup raw vegetables with 2 tablespoons natural peanut butter

WEEK 4 PREP LIST

- Chop fruit and vegetables for meals, snacks, and side dishes.
- Make Hash Brown Vegetable Breakfast Casserole (page 91).

- Hard-boil 3 eggs.
- Prep Apple Cinnamon Overnight Oats (page 81).
- Make Dark Chocolate Walnut Bars (page 83).

- Make Coconut Date Energy Bites (page 191), if using for snacks.

WEEK 4 SHOPPING LIST

Produce

Apple (1)

Avocados (5)

Basil (1 container)

Cabbage, Napa (1 head)

Cabbage, red (1 cup shredded or 1 small head)

Cauliflower (1 head)

Carrots (½ cup shredded or 2)

Cilantro (1 bunch)

Coleslaw mix (1 [10-ounce] bag)

Cucumber, English (1)

Dill or chives (1 container)

Fruit, fresh (8 pieces or 8 chopped cups)

Garlic (1 head)

Ginger (1 piece)

Kale (1 bunch, or 2 cups chopped)

Leek (1)

Lemon (1)

Lettuce, romaine (2 to 3 heads)

Limes (2)

Onions, yellow (3)

Peaches (3)

Pepper, jalapeño (1)

Peppers, bell (2)

Scallions (2)

Spinach, baby (6 to 8 cups)

Strawberries (1 quart)

Sweet potatoes (2)

Thyme (1 container)

Tomato (1)

Tomatoes, cherry (2 pints)

Vegetables, raw (baby carrots, cucumber, bell pepper, and others) (4 cups)

Dairy

Buttermilk, low fat (1 small carton)

Cheese, feta (½ cup)

Cheese, Mexican-style, shredded (1 cup)

Cheese, Parmesan, grated (¼ cup)

Cheese, sharp Cheddar, shredded (2 cups)

Eggs, large (30)

Milk, skim (½ gallon)

Yogurt, nonfat plain Greek (1 [32-ounce] tub)

Meat, Poultry, and Fish

Beef, ground (90/10) (1½ pounds)

Chicken, ground (2 pounds)

Chicken thighs, boneless, skinless (1 pound)

Pork, sirloin roast (2 pounds)

Salmon (2 pounds)

Canned/Dried Goods

Beans, kidney, no salt added (2 [15-ounce] cans)

Oranges, mandarin (1 [8-ounce] can)

Tomato paste, no salt added (2 tablespoons)

Tomatoes, crushed, no salt added (1 [32-ounce] can)

Frozen

Edamame, shelled (½ cup)

Potatoes, hash brown (3 cups)

Grains

Buns, sandwich, whole wheat, slider size (8)

Pasta, orecchiette (12 ounces)

Tortillas, whole wheat, 8-inch (9)

Pantry Items

Almonds, sliced (½ cup)

Oil, coconut (1 small jar)

YOUR EXERCISE ROUTINE

Cardio workouts should be 30 minutes in duration, but you can work up to this length if you are a beginner. Strength workouts should include 3 to 4 sets of 8 to 10 repetitions of each exercise where applicable. In the case of static core exercises such as the plank, work toward holding the movements for longer each week.

My Exercise Routine

The following is your exercise plan for the week. Fill in the table with the cardio and strength-training exercises (pages 33–37) you plan to do.

M	T	W	TH	F	SAT	S
Cardio:	Cardio:	R E S T	Cardio:	R E S T	Cardio:	R E S T
	Core		Core			
	Lower Body		Lower Body			
	Upper Body		Upper Body			
	Full Body		Full Body			

YOUR HABIT TRACKER

The habit tracker is an optional but very useful tool to help you keep tabs on some of the important health behaviors that are encouraged throughout the book. Sleeping eight hours a night, meditation, and eating your recommended daily servings of vegetables are all very important habits that you could potentially choose to track using this helpful tool.

My Habit Tracker

It's important to make healthy lifestyle choices in addition to dietary changes. Create a list of healthy habits you want to maintain over the next four weeks and mark the days when you succeed.

HABIT	M	T	W	TH	F	SAT	S
Drank 8 glasses of water	X		X	X		X	

Beyond 28 Days

Congratulations on completing the first 28 days of the rest of your life. That's exactly how I encourage you to look at it. You've taken serious strides toward your health goals and should be proud of all that you've accomplished thus far. While one chapter has come to a close, your commitment to healthier living has hopefully only just begun. Whatever your ultimate goals are, this section will offer you some valuable insights that will go a long way in helping you achieve them.

MAINTAINING YOUR PRIORITIES

By following through with your best effort in the last 28 days, you've made a real and tangible commitment to your health. But this is only the beginning. It's up to you to take that next critical step and transition away from a short-term plan to a long-term lifestyle.

With that in mind, now is the time to acknowledge three very important realities:

Your next 280 days are more important than the last 28. The one thing about healthy eating and exercise is that the more you do it, the more benefit you get out of it. Your 28-day plan was never meant to be a quick fix or magic-bullet solution. It was meant to offer you a pathway to healthier eating for life.

There will be ups and downs. What I always tell my clients is that I care much more about what they do most of the time than what they do once in a while. I promise you, life will get in the way of your best intentions when it comes to diet and exercise. I'm also telling you right now, it doesn't matter. Live your life in the way that makes you happy, and always keep in mind that a few meals out with friends, or that piece of cake you love, will never truly detract from the balanced diet you enjoy the rest of the time.

You are going to be okay. The DASH diet style is considered among the easiest eating patterns to follow for good reason. It includes a wide variety of foods and restricts none. If you have enjoyed yourself on the first 28 days of this program, there's no reason why you won't enjoy yourself on the next 337. Even if there are periods of time where a balanced diet seems beyond you, know that you have a strong foundation to return to, and you've already proven to yourself that you can do it.

TAKING THE "WORK" OUT OF "WORKOUTS"

For the sake of your good health, my hope is that you will be able to develop a regular exercise routine that builds on some of the structure you were provided in your 28-day plan. Even so, it's safe to say that despite your best efforts and intentions, keeping up a diligent and structured exercise routine can be challenging. You have a great foundation to work with, but you also have the flexibility and freedom to break a sweat, expend some energy, and enjoy the health benefits of exercise through different types of activities, especially those that take place outdoors.

Great examples include:

- Riding a bike

- Hiking

- Mowing the lawn

- Chopping wood

- Shoveling snow

- Carrying your own clubs while golfing

- Tennis

Remember, a major key to your success when it comes to exercise is finding something you enjoy and can do regularly and safely. Don't be fooled into thinking that exercise takes place only in a gym or within the sampling of exercises that you've been provided in this book. There are a lot of options out there. There will be days where working out indoors is the last thing you want to do, so take it outside if you are able. In addition to being great forms of exercise, activities that involve you being outdoors in nature offer proven benefits to your mood and mental health as well.

ACHIEVING LONG-TERM SUCCESS

Track your sleep habits. I've spoken at length about the important connection between sufficient sleep and good health. Consistent sleep is incredibly important and something that can get away from you if you don't stay on top of it. Taking the time to track your weekly sleeping habits using a smartphone or journal can be a gentle and valuable reminder to aim for that eight hours most nights.

Share your goals with friends and family. If you haven't already, consider making it a point to share your healthy eating goals and ambitions with your friends and family. One of the most famous and well-known models of behavior change says that when people share their ambitions to change with those closest to them, it helps them on their path to success. The support and understanding of your loved ones will be invaluable for your health in the long term.

Spend time with like-minded people. Are there people in your life who are living a healthy, active lifestyle? They have probably gone through similar changes and may be able to offer you valuable insights to help you stay on track with your healthy eating goals. Consider reaching out to at least one such person in your life, as you will be invaluable resources to one another.

Learn to accept setbacks. Guess what? Things aren't always going to go as planned. It's much easier to do something for 28 days than it is for 280 days, so make sure you embrace the fact that for some days, weeks, or even months your overall eating pattern may not be as balanced as the ones before, but that does not detract from the good work you've done, nor does it take away from the good work you can continue to do.

Create an environment conducive to success. When it comes to your dietary choices, your environment is represented by your kitchen, fridge, and pantry. In order for those environments to be conducive to your success, they must be well stocked with the healthy foods that will help you fulfill your DASH diet goals. Getting into the habit of creating grocery lists and setting a specific day each week for grocery shopping will help facilitate this goal.

Set sustainable exercise goals. Although you may not stick to the exact routine provided in your 28-day plan, try your best to set weekly exercise goals in terms of both the duration and number of days you intend to exercise. Remember that it does not always need to be a gym workout; it's the total amount of exercise you get per week that's important. Aim for 120 to 150 minutes weekly, per CDC recommendations.

Keep track of how many meals you eat out. Eating and drinking out with friends, family, or even alone are all completely normal parts of life. It's also important to accept that meals out tend to be higher in sodium, cost, and calories. Find a number of meals out a week that balances your social life, happiness, and overall nutrition goals. That number will be different for different people.

BONUS MENUS

As you move past the initial 28-day plan, we hope you have gained the skills and confidence to build your own plan that works with your lifestyle. Because our goal is to help you achieve a smooth transition into building your own plan, we've provided a supplemental two-week menu with new recipes and meal ideas. Congratulations on your continued success!

Bonus Week 1

Monday

Breakfast

6 ounces nonfat fruit-flavored Greek yogurt

1 cup or medium piece fresh fruit

½ cup high-fiber cereal

Lunch

Tuscan Chicken & Kale Soup (page 108)

1 slice whole-grain baguette

Dinner

Chili Garlic-Crusted Pork Chops (page 182)

1 small baked potato with 1 tablespoon plain Greek yogurt

1 cup cooked vegetables

Snacks

2 to 3; midmorning, midafternoon, and evening

Tuesday

Breakfast

Whole-grain English muffin, toasted

1 fried egg

1 slice low-sodium cheese

1 cup or medium piece fresh fruit

Lunch

Leftover Tuscan Chicken & Kale Soup (page 108)

1 slice whole-grain baguette

Dinner

Mexican-Style Turkey Stuffed Peppers (page 164)

1 cup or medium piece fresh fruit

Snacks

2 to 3; midmorning, midafternoon, and evening

Wednesday

Breakfast

6 ounces nonfat fruit-flavored Greek yogurt

1 cup or medium piece fresh fruit

½ cup high-fiber cereal

Lunch

Leftover Mexican-Style Turkey Stuffed Peppers (page 164)

1 cup or medium piece fresh fruit

Dinner

Gnocchi with Tomato Basil Sauce (page 142)

Green salad with 2 tablespoons dressing

Snacks

2 to 3; midmorning, midafternoon, and evening

Thursday

Breakfast

Whole-grain English muffin, toasted

1 fried egg

1 slice low-sodium cheese

1 cup or medium piece fresh fruit

Lunch

Leftover Gnocchi with Tomato Basil Sauce (page 142)

Green salad with 2 tablespoons dressing

Dinner

Classic Pot Roast (page 178)

1 cup or medium piece fresh fruit

Snacks

2 to 3; midmorning, midafternoon, and evening

Friday

Breakfast

Protein bar

1 cup or medium piece fresh fruit

Lunch

Leftover Classic Pot Roast (page 178)

1 cup or medium piece fresh fruit

Dinner

Shrimp Pasta Primavera (page 156)

Green salad with 2 tablespoons dressing

Snacks

2 to 3; midmorning, midafternoon, and evening

Saturday

Breakfast

Roasted Red Pepper & Pesto Omelet (page 88)

1 cup or medium piece fresh fruit

Lunch

Chipotle Chicken & Caramelized Onion Panini (page 118)

½ cup raw vegetables

Dinner

Lentil Avocado Tacos (page 138)

Grilled Corn & Edamame Succotash (page 196)

Dessert

½ cup frozen yogurt or ice cream

1 cup fresh fruit

Snacks

1 to 2; midmorning and midafternoon

Sunday

Breakfast

Sweet Potato Pancakes with Maple Yogurt (page 92)

1 cup or medium piece fresh fruit

Lunch

Leftover Lentil Avocado Tacos (page 138)

Leftover Grilled Corn & Edamame Succotash (page 196)

Dinner

Beef & Vegetable Stir-Fry (page 175)

Dessert

½ cup frozen yogurt or ice cream

1 cup fresh fruit

Snacks

1 to 2; midmorning and midafternoon

Suggested Snacks

Hummus & Vegetable–Stuffed Collard Wrap (page 124)

¼ cup nuts with 1 cup raw vegetables

Medium piece fruit with 1 tablespoon natural peanut butter

6 ounces nonfat fruit-flavored Greek yogurt with ½ cup fresh fruit

1 cup bell pepper slices with 2 tablespoons hummus

Bonus Week 2

Monday

Breakfast

6 ounces nonfat fruit-flavored Greek yogurt

1 cup or medium piece fresh fruit

½ cup high-fiber cereal

Lunch

White Bean, Chicken & Green Chili (page 112)

7 to 8 whole-grain corn tortilla chips

Dinner

Spinach & Artichoke Grilled Cheese (page 117)

½ cup raw vegetables

Snacks

2 to 3; midmorning, midafternoon, and evening

Tuesday

Breakfast

Whole-grain English muffin, toasted

1 fried egg

1 slice low-sodium cheese

1 cup or medium piece fresh fruit

Lunch

Leftover White Bean, Chicken & Green Chili (page 112)

7 to 8 whole-grain corn tortilla chips

Dinner

Peanut Vegetable Pad Thai (page 126)

1 cup or medium piece fresh fruit

Snacks

2 to 3; midmorning, midafternoon, and evening

Wednesday

Breakfast

6 ounces nonfat fruit-flavored Greek yogurt

1 cup or medium piece fresh fruit

½ cup high-fiber cereal

Lunch

Leftover Peanut Vegetable Pad Thai (page 126)

1 cup or medium piece fresh fruit

Dinner

Italian Stuffed Portobello Mushroom Burgers (page 140)

Green salad with 2 tablespoons dressing

Snacks

2 to 3; midmorning, midafternoon, and evening

Thursday

Breakfast

Whole-grain English muffin, toasted

1 fried egg

1 slice low-sodium cheese

1 cup or medium piece fresh fruit

Lunch

Leftover Italian Stuffed Portobello Mushroom Burgers (page 140)

Green salad with 2 tablespoons dressing

Dinner

Slow Cooker Pork Carnitas (page 183)

1 cup or medium piece fresh fruit

Snacks

2 to 3; midmorning, midafternoon, and evening

Friday

Breakfast

Protein bar

1 cup or medium piece fresh fruit

Lunch

Leftover Slow Cooker Pork Carnitas (page 183)

1 cup or medium piece fresh fruit

Dinner

Almond-Crusted Tuna Cakes (page 151)

Maple Mustard Brussels Sprouts with Toasted Walnuts (page 198)

Snacks

2 to 3; midmorning, midafternoon, and evening

Saturday

Breakfast

Roasted Red Pepper & Pesto Omelet (page 88)

1 cup or medium piece fresh fruit

Lunch

Leftover Almond-Crusted Tuna Cakes (page 151)

Leftover Maple Mustard Brussels Sprouts with Toasted Walnuts (page 198)

Dinner

Creamy Pumpkin Pasta (page 143)

Green salad with 2 tablespoons dressing

Dessert

½ cup frozen yogurt or ice cream

1 cup fresh fruit

Snacks

1 to 2; midmorning and midafternoon

Sunday

Breakfast

Peanut Butter & Banana Oatmeal (page 82)

1 hard-boiled egg

Lunch

Leftover Creamy Pumpkin Pasta (page 143)

Green salad with 2 tablespoons dressing

Dinner

Taco-Stuffed Sweet Potatoes (page 176)

1 cup or medium piece fresh fruit

Dessert

½ cup frozen yogurt or ice cream

1 cup fresh fruit

Snacks

1 to 2; midmorning and midafternoon

Suggested Snacks

Hummus & Vegetable–Stuffed Collard Wrap (page 124)

¼ cup nuts with 1 cup raw vegetables

Medium piece fruit with 1 tablespoon natural peanut butter

6 ounces nonfat fruit-flavored Greek yogurt with ½ cup fresh fruit

1 cup bell pepper slices with 2 tablespoons hummus

Make Your Own Weekly Menu

Being able to design your own weekly menu with confidence is a sign of progression within the confines of the DASH diet but also demonstrates mastery over your understanding of the recommended food groups and serving sizes. You've probably enjoyed many of the recipes that this book has to offer, but now is your chance to go ahead and try something new, which may include spin-offs or variations of your favorite dishes. Keep your personal DASH diet serving-size guidelines in mind, and use the Healthy Plate on page 18 for further guidance in terms of how to structure your meals.

	BREAKFAST	LUNCH	DINNER	SNACK
Monday				
Tuesday				
Wednesday				
Thursday				
Friday				
Saturday				
Sunday				

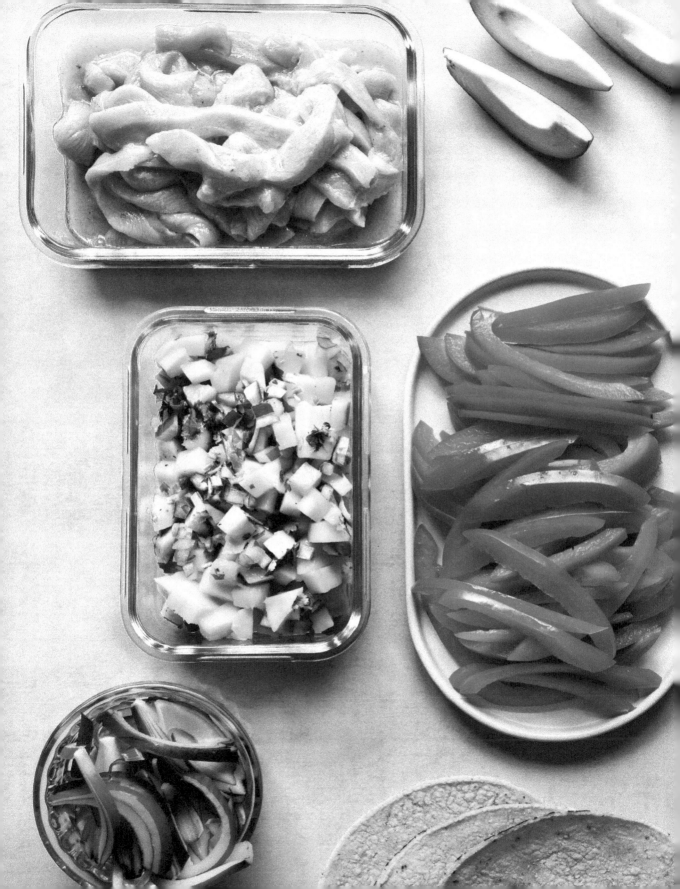

PART TWO

The Recipes

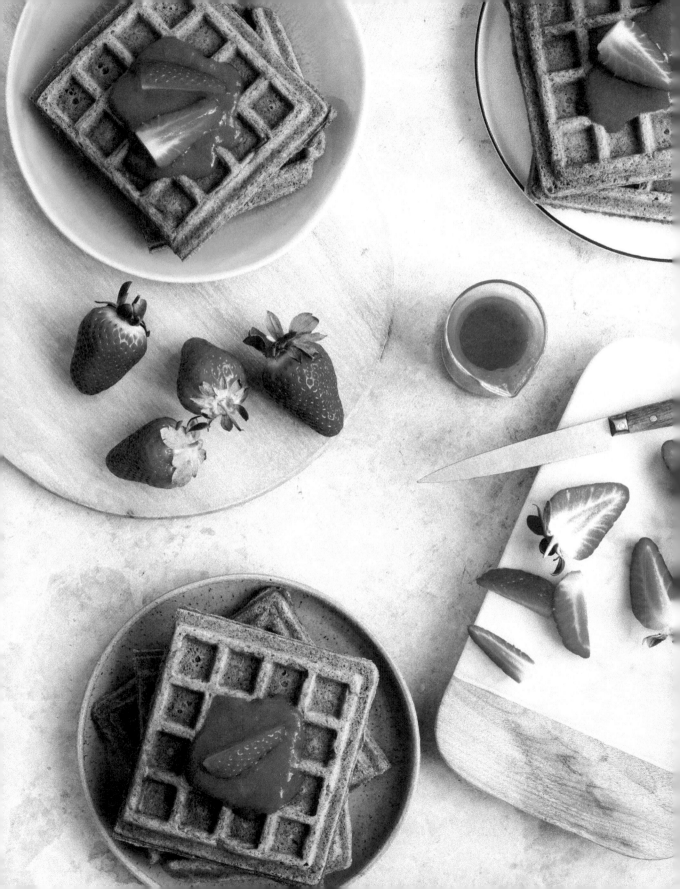

5

Breakfasts and Smoothies

Mango Pineapple Green Smoothie

VEGETARIAN • UNDER 30 MINUTES

SERVES 2 PREP TIME: 5 MINUTES

Head to the tropics with this smoothie. The greens add beautiful color and nutrients without overpowering the flavors of mango, pineapple, and orange, and the Greek yogurt adds protein to keep you full and satisfied for hours.

1 cup frozen mango chunks

1 cup frozen pineapple chunks

1 cup fresh spinach or kale

1¼ cups orange juice

½ cup nonfat plain or vanilla
   Greek yogurt

1 tablespoon ground flaxseed

1 teaspoon granulated stevia

1. Place all of the ingredients in the pitcher of a blender. Purée until smooth.
2. Serve immediately.

SUBSTITUTION TIP: Any milk (cow's, almond, soy, coconut) can be used in this recipe instead of the yogurt.

COOKING TIP: Choose calcium and vitamin D-fortified orange juice, if possible.

VARIATION TIP: Replace mango and pineapple with mixed berries for a green berry smoothie.

MAKE IT A MEAL: Add 1 to 2 scoops protein powder to make this smoothie a protein-packed meal.

PER SERVING: Total Calories: 213; Total Fat: 2g; Saturated Fat: 0g; Cholesterol: 2.5mg; Sodium: 44mg; Potassium: 582mg; Total Carbohydrate: 43g; Fiber: 4g; Sugars: 34g; Protein: 9g

Morning Glory Smoothie

SERVES 2   PREP TIME: 10 MINUTES

We've taken the classic flavors of apple, walnut, carrot, and coconut, and put them into a smoothie that is packed with fiber, vitamins, and minerals so you can start your day off right.

1 cup nonfat milk

½ cup 100% apple juice

2 tablespoons chopped walnuts

2 tablespoons unsweetened coconut flakes

2 frozen bananas

1 small carrot, peeled and chopped

½ teaspoon ground cinnamon

½ teaspoon pure vanilla extract

½ teaspoon granulated stevia

1 to 2 cups ice cubes

1. Place the milk, apple juice, walnuts, and coconut flakes in the pitcher of a blender. Let sit 5 minutes.

2. Add the frozen bananas, carrot, cinnamon, vanilla extract, stevia, and ice cubes to the pitcher. Purée until smooth.

3. Serve immediately.

SUBSTITUTION TIP: Any milk (cow's, almond, soy, coconut) can be used in this recipe.

COOKING TIP: Before freezing bananas, peel, slice, and place them in sealed zip-top bags.

VARIATION TIP: Omit the apple juice and add 1 apple, peeled, cored, and roughly chopped for a boost of fiber.

MAKE IT A MEAL: Add 1 to 2 scoops protein powder to make this smoothie a protein-packed meal.

PER SERVING: Total Calories: 276; Total Fat: 8g; Saturated Fat: 4g; Cholesterol: 2mg; Sodium: 72mg; Potassium: 708mg; Total Carbohydrate: 46g; Fiber: 6g; Sugars: 30g; Protein: 6g

Peach Avocado Smoothie

VEGETARIAN • UNDER 30 MINUTES

SERVES 2   PREP TIME: 15 MINUTES

Avocados make the perfect accompaniment to a fruit smoothie because they add a rich, creamy texture while providing fiber and heart-healthy fat. Adding flax or chia seeds gives a slight nutty flavor with a boost of omega-3 fatty acids.

1½ cups frozen peaches

1½ cups nonfat milk

1 cup nonfat plain or vanilla
    Greek yogurt

1 avocado, peeled and pitted

1 tablespoon ground flaxseed

1½ teaspoons granulated stevia

1 teaspoon pure vanilla extract

1 to 2 cups ice cubes

1. Combine all the ingredients in a blender. Purée until smooth.
2. Serve immediately.

SUBSTITUTION TIP: Any milk (cow's, almond, soy, coconut) can be used in this recipe.

COOKING TIP: To ripen an avocado quicker, store it in a brown paper bag in a dry, cool place.

VARIATION TIP: Replace out peaches with mango, pineapple, or berries.

MAKE IT A MEAL: Add 1 to 2 scoops protein powder to make this smoothie a protein-packed meal.

PER SERVING: Total Calories: 323; Total Fat: 15g; Saturated Fat: 2g; Cholesterol: 9mg; Sodium: 142mg; Potassium: 1,186mg; Total Carbohydrate: 32g; Fiber: 8g; Sugars: 21g; Protein: 21g

Apple Cinnamon Overnight Oats

VEGETARIAN

SERVES 2 **PREP TIME: 15 MINUTES** PLUS AT LEAST 4 HOURS REFRIGERATION

This breakfast is a mash-up of sweet morning oatmeal and freshly baked apple pie. Besides their classic flavor combination of apples and cinnamon, the best part about these overnight oats is that they're quick to make, use ingredients most of us have on hand, and are prep-ahead, making weekday mornings stress-free and delicious.

1 cup old-fashioned rolled oats

2 tablespoons chia seeds or ground flaxseed

1¼ cups nonfat milk

½ tablespoon ground cinnamon

2 teaspoons honey or pure maple syrup

½ teaspoon pure vanilla extract

Dash of kosher or sea salt

1 apple, diced

1. Divide the oats, chia seeds or ground flaxseed, milk, cinnamon, honey or maple syrup, vanilla extract, and salt into two Mason jars. Place the lids tightly on top and shake until thoroughly combined.

2. Remove the lids and add half of the diced apple to each jar. Sprinkle with additional cinnamon, if desired. Place the lids tightly back on the jars and refrigerate for at least 4 hours or overnight.

3. You can store the overnight oats in single-serve containers in the refrigerator for up to 3 days.

SUBSTITUTION TIP: Any milk (cow's, almond, soy, coconut) can be used in this recipe.

COOKING TIP: If you don't have Mason jars, simply whisk the overnight oat mixture in a bowl and transfer to containers with airtight lids.

VARIATION TIP: Replace out the cinnamon and apples with mango and coconut for tropical overnight oats.

MAKE IT A MEAL: Serve with cooked chicken sausage or stir in 2 tablespoons of nut butter for a complete meal.

PER SERVING: Total Calories: 339; Total Fat: 8g; Saturated Fat: 1g; Cholesterol: 3mg; Sodium: 66mg; Potassium: 363mg; Total Carbohydrate: 60g; Fiber: 12g; Sugars: 24g; Protein: 13g

Peanut Butter & Banana Oatmeal

VEGETARIAN • MEAL-IN-ONE • UNDER 30 MINUTES

SERVES 6   PREP TIME: 10 MINUTES   COOK TIME: 10 MINUTES

Peanut butter and bananas are a classic combination. Their flavors and textures work well in classic maple-sweetened oatmeal. You can prep and cook this recipe in advance and eat it cold or warm it up on weekdays for a quick and simple yet rich and luxurious breakfast.

2 cups old-fashioned rolled oats

3½ cups water

½ cup natural peanut butter

3 tablespoons pure maple syrup

½ tablespoons ground cinnamon

1 teaspoon pure vanilla extract

½ teaspoon kosher or sea salt

½ cup nonfat milk

2 ripe bananas, peeled and sliced

SUBSTITUTION TIP: Steel-cut oats can be used instead of old-fashioned rolled.

COOKING TIP: Sauté the banana slices in a small amount of oil for a caramelized, sweet finish.

VARIATION TIP: Use any nut butter or fruit for this recipe to change things up.

PER SERVING: Total Calories: 298; Total Fat: 13g; Saturated Fat: 2g; Cholesterol: 0mg; Sodium: 304mg; Potassium: 178mg; Total Carbohydrate: 39g; Fiber: 5g; Sugars: 15g; Protein: 9g

1. Pour the oats and water into a medium saucepan and bring to a simmer. Cook for about 5 minutes, stirring frequently, until the oats are soft.

2. Remove from the heat and stir in the peanut butter, maple syrup, cinnamon, vanilla extract, and salt until combined.

3. Divide the oatmeal into bowls and top with the milk and sliced bananas.

4. Place leftovers in airtight microwaveable containers and refrigerate for up to 5 days. Reheat by microwaving on high 1½ to 2 minutes.

Dark Chocolate Walnut Bars

SERVES 12   PREP TIME: 15 MINUTES PLUS AT LEAST 2 HOURS REFRIGERATION

To reap the antioxidant benefits of dark chocolate, be sure to choose chocolate that is at least 60 percent cacao. The walnuts are also packed with nutrition, providing omega-3 fatty acids, fiber, and protein, which are all important for overall health.

2 cups chopped walnuts

2 cups unsweetened shredded coconut

12 pitted Medjool dates

½ cup dark cocoa powder

¼ cup melted coconut oil

¼ cup dark chocolate chips

3 tablespoons honey

1 teaspoon pure vanilla extract

1. Line an 8-by-8-inch baking dish with parchment paper.

2. Place all the ingredients in the bowl of a food processor and pulse until a sticky dough forms. Transfer the dough to the prepared baking dish and spread the dough evenly using the back of a spoon. Cover with plastic wrap and refrigerate for at least 2 hours, until set.

3. Lift the edges of the parchment paper and transfer the bars to a cutting board. Cut into 12 equal-size squares.

4. Store the bars in sealed plastic bags. They can be stored at room temperature for up to 2 weeks and frozen for up to 2 months.

SUBSTITUTION TIP: If you don't have dates, you can replace them with raisins or prunes.

COOKING TIP: Be sure to use melted coconut oil versus another oil, like canola or olive. Coconut oil is a saturated fat and will harden at room temperature or when refrigerated, which holds the bars together.

VARIATION TIP: Replace walnuts with almonds or cashews.

PER SERVING: Total Calories: 375; Total Fat: 29g; Saturated Fat: 14g; Cholesterol: 0mg; Sodium: 50mg; Potassium: 256mg; Total Carbohydrate: 34g; Fiber: 6g; Sugars: 24g; Protein: 5g

Blueberry Date Muffins

SERVES 12   PREP TIME: 15 MINUTES   COOK TIME: 25 MINUTES

These date- and blueberry-packed muffins are light and fluffy, yet contain high-fiber ingredients to make for a filling snack or part of a meal. The yogurt provides a boost of probiotics while moistening the lower-fat muffins, and the dates provide sweetness without much added sugar.

1¼ cups whole-wheat flour or whole-wheat pastry flour

½ cup old-fashioned rolled oats

1 teaspoon baking powder

1 teaspoon baking soda

¼ teaspoon kosher or sea salt

¼ teaspoon ground cinnamon

¼ cup oil

¼ cup dark brown sugar

2 large eggs

1 teaspoon pure vanilla extract

⅔ cup milk or nonfat plain Greek yogurt

1 cup frozen or fresh blueberries

8 pitted Medjool dates, chopped

1. Preheat the oven to 350°F. Line a 12-cup muffin tin with muffin liners.

2. In a bowl, stir together the flour, oats, baking powder, baking soda, salt, and cinnamon until combined.

3. In a separate bowl, whisk together the oil and brown sugar until fluffy. Whisk in the eggs, one at a time, until well beaten. Whisk in the vanilla extract and milk or yogurt until combined.

4. Add the flour mixture to the wet ingredients and stir until just combined, then gently fold in the blueberries and dates.

5. Evenly spoon the batter into each muffin liner, filling almost all the way to the top. Bake for 25 minutes, until a toothpick inserted into the center comes out clean. Let slightly cool before removing from the muffin tin.

6. Store the cooled muffins in sealed plastic bags. They can be stored at room temperature for up to a week or can be frozen for up to 2 months.

SUBSTITUTION TIP: Whole-wheat pastry flour is the perfect substitute for all-purpose or whole-wheat flour. It's light but packed with fiber, and will preserve the texture of a delicate muffin.

COOKING TIP: To save time, look for prechopped dates in the dried fruit or baking section of your grocery store.

VARIATION TIP: Leave out the blueberries and mix in dark chocolate chips.

MAKE IT A MEAL: These muffins make the perfect snack. To make them into a meal, serve with scrambled eggs, or chicken sausage and a side of fruit.

PER SERVING: Total Calories: 180; Total Fat: 6g; Saturated Fat: 1g; Cholesterol: 35mg; Sodium: 172mg; Potassium: 186mg; Total Carbohydrate: 30g; Fiber: 3g; Sugars: 17g; Protein: 4g

Broccoli Cheese Egg Muffins

VEGETARIAN · MEAL-IN-ONE

SERVES 4 (3 EGG MUFFINS EACH)   PREP TIME: 15 MINUTES   COOK TIME: 30 MINUTES

These mini frittatas are loaded with broccoli and Cheddar cheese. The flavor provided by the onion, garlic, and mustard makes them anything but boring. You can prep them in advance and eat high-protein, satisfying breakfasts all week.

1 tablespoon olive oil

1 small head broccoli, chopped into bite-size florets (about 4 cups)

8 large eggs

¼ cup nonfat milk

1 teaspoon onion powder

1 teaspoon garlic powder

¼ teaspoon kosher or sea salt

½ teaspoon ground black pepper

½ teaspoon dried mustard powder

1 cup shredded Cheddar cheese, divided

Cooking spray

1. Heat the olive oil in a medium skillet over medium heat. Add the broccoli and sauté 4 to 5 minutes, until soft.

2. In a large mixing bowl, whisk together the eggs, milk, onion powder, garlic powder, salt, black pepper, and mustard powder. Fold in the sautéed broccoli and half of the Cheddar cheese.

3. Coat a 12-cup muffin tin with cooking spray. Evenly distribute the egg mixture into each cup. Sprinkle with the remaining Cheddar cheese. Bake for 18 to 22 minutes, until the eggs are set.

4. Let the muffins slightly cool before removing from the tin.

5. Place the egg muffins in microwaveable airtight containers and refrigerate for up to 5 days or freeze for up to 2 months. Reheat in the microwave for 1 to 2 minutes on high, until heated through.

SUBSTITUTION TIP: Plain nonfat Greek yogurt can be substituted for the milk in this recipe for an added boost of protein.

COOKING TIP: Batches of sautéed broccoli can be prepared in advance and used in this recipe or as a side dish for other meals.

VARIATION TIP: Roasted or sautéed asparagus, bell peppers, or mushrooms are great substitutes for the broccoli.

PER SERVING: Total Calories: 316; Total Fat: 23g; Saturated Fat: 11g; Cholesterol: 447mg; Sodium: 496mg; Potassium: 323mg; Total Carbohydrate: 7g; Fiber: 3g; Sugars: 2g; Protein: 21g

Greek Breakfast Scramble

SERVES 4   PREP TIME: 10 MINUTES   COOK TIME: 10 MINUTES

Whole eggs provide protein, vitamin D, and choline, an essential nutrient for brain and heart health. When slow-scrambled with a rainbow of vegetables, they make for a simple and flavorful breakfast that is ready in no time.

1 tablespoon olive oil

1 pint grape or cherry tomatoes, quartered

2 cups chopped kale

2 garlic cloves, peeled and minced

8 large eggs

¼ teaspoon kosher or sea salt

¼ teaspoon ground black pepper

¼ cup crumbled feta

¼ cup flat-leaf Italian parsley, chopped

1. Heat the olive oil in a large nonstick skillet over medium heat. Add the tomatoes and kale. Sauté for 2 to 3 minutes, until the kale and tomatoes are slightly soft. Stir in the garlic. Reduce the skillet heat to low.

2. In a medium bowl, whisk together the eggs, salt, and black pepper. Pour the egg mixture into the skillet, slowly folding the eggs until fluffy and scrambled. Remove from the heat and fold in the feta and parsley.

3. Store the scramble in microwaveable airtight containers and refrigerate for up to 5 days. Reheat by microwaving on high for 60 to 90 seconds, until heated through.

SUBSTITUTION TIP: Use egg whites for a lower-fat, higher-protein scramble.

COOKING TIP: Cook eggs on low heat to avoid them becoming dry and rubbery. Constantly and slowly fold the eggs with a spatula until they're light and fluffy.

VARIATION TIP: Use chopped spinach, mustard greens, or collard greens instead of kale.

MAKE IT A MEAL: Serve with a slice of whole-wheat toast or fresh fruit.

PER SERVING: Total Calories: 222; Total Fat: 15g; Saturated Fat: 5g; Cholesterol: 427mg; Sodium: 383mg; Potassium: 195mg; Total Carbohydrate: 7g; Fiber: 1g; Sugars: 0g; Protein: 15g

Roasted Red Pepper & Pesto Omelet

SERVES 4   PREP TIME: 10 MINUTES   COOK TIME: 20 MINUTES

You can put almost any vegetable in an omelet, and this variation takes the traditional omelet to the next level with roasted red peppers and pesto. Make the pesto at home with fresh basil and spinach so you can instantly add flavor to many dishes with one sauce.

8 large eggs

¼ cup Basil Pesto (page 212) or store-bought pesto

¼ teaspoon ground black pepper

⅛ teaspoon kosher or sea salt

Cooking spray

½ cup baby spinach leaves

½ cup jarred roasted red peppers, chopped

¾ cup shredded white Cheddar cheese

1. Heat a large nonstick skillet over medium-low heat.

2. In a medium bowl, whisk together the eggs, pesto, black pepper, and salt until thoroughly combined.

3. Coat the skillet with the cooking spray. Add ¼ of the spinach and stir until slightly wilted. Pour in ¼ of the egg mixture. Let cook for 2 to 3 minutes, until the egg is almost set. Place ¼ of the roasted red peppers and cheese in the center of the omelet. Fold the omelet in half. Place a lid on top and cook for 1 to 2 minutes, until the cheese is melted.

4. Repeat step 3 with the remaining ingredients to make 4 omelets total.

5. Store the omelets in microwaveable airtight containers and refrigerate for up to 5 days. Reheat by microwaving on high for 2 minutes, until heated through.

SUBSTITUTION TIP: Use the Basil Pesto (page 212) to lower the sodium content, as jarred pesto tends to be quite high in sodium.

COOKING TIP: Pour leftover pesto into ice cube trays and freeze them to have home-made pesto anytime.

VARIATION TIP: Replace roasted red peppers with kalamata olives or artichokes.

MAKE IT A MEAL: Serve with a slice of whole-wheat toast or a side of fruit.

PER SERVING: Total Calories: 314; Total Fat: 24g; Saturated Fat: 9g; Cholesterol: 444mg; Sodium: 499mg; Potassium: 0mg; Total Carbohydrate: 5g; Fiber: 1g; Sugars: 1g; Protein: 19g

Mushroom Thyme Frittata

VEGETARIAN · MEAL-IN-ONE

SERVES 6   PREP TIME: 15 MINUTES   COOK TIME: 25 MINUTES

With flavors of mushrooms, thyme, and Swiss cheese, this simple make-ahead meal is perfect to reheat during the week with no fuss. Replace the mushrooms with roasted asparagus for a springtime favorite.

12 large eggs

½ cup nonfat plain Greek yogurt

1 tablespoon balsamic vinegar

¾ teaspoon kosher or sea salt

¼ teaspoon ground black pepper

1½ cups shredded Swiss cheese, divided

3 tablespoons olive oil

1 large shallot, peeled and thinly sliced

2 scallions, thinly sliced

2 cups sliced mushrooms

2 teaspoons fresh thyme leaves, chopped

1. Preheat the oven to 375°F.

2. In a large mixing bowl, whisk together the eggs, Greek yogurt, balsamic vinegar, salt, and black pepper and half of the shredded Swiss cheese until thoroughly combined.

3. Heat the olive oil in a large oven-safe nonstick skillet over medium heat. Add the shallots, scallions, and mushrooms and sauté 4 to 5 minutes, until the mushrooms are soft. Stir in the thyme.

4. Pour the egg mixture into the skillet with the mushroom mixture and cook 4 to 5 minutes, until the bottom starts to set. Top with the remaining shredded cheese and transfer to the oven. Bake for 15 minutes, until the egg is set.

5. Remove the frittata from the oven and let slightly cool, then slice into 6 wedges.

6. Store the frittata slices in microwaveable airtight containers and refrigerate for up to 5 days. Reheat by microwaving on high for 60 to 90 seconds, until heated through.

SUBSTITUTION TIP: For a lower-fat frittata, use egg whites instead of whole eggs.

COOKING TIP: If you don't have fresh thyme, use 1 teaspoon dried instead.

VARIATION TIP: Replace mushrooms with roasted asparagus.

PER SERVING: Total Calories: 333; Total Fat: 25g; Saturated Fat: 10g; Cholesterol: 448mg; Sodium: 503mg; Potassium: 142mg; Total Carbohydrate: 4g; Fiber: 0g; Sugars: 2g; Protein: 22g

Roasted Root Vegetable Hash

VEGETARIAN · MEAL-IN-ONE

SERVES 4   PREP TIME: 20 MINUTES   COOK TIME: 40 MINUTES

Roasted vegetable hash is a simple and flavorful way to get in several servings of vegetables while satisfying your cravings for something savory. Top the hash with runny-yolk eggs for a dreamy dish that's reminiscent of an upscale restaurant breakfast.

Cooking spray

2 small sweet potatoes, peeled and cubed

2 parsnips, peeled and sliced

1 red onion, thinly sliced

2 tablespoons olive oil

½ tablespoon balsamic vinegar

¼ teaspoon kosher or sea salt

½ teaspoon ground black pepper

¼ teaspoon crushed red pepper flakes

8 Perfectly Poached Eggs (page 210)

1. Preheat the oven to 400°F. Coat a baking sheet with the cooking spray.

2. Place the sweet potatoes, parsnips, and red onion on the greased baking sheet. Drizzle with the olive oil and balsamic vinegar and sprinkle with the salt, black pepper, and crushed red pepper flakes. Toss to coat.

3. Roast for 35 to 40 minutes, until vegetables are fork tender and crispy on the outside.

4. Serve with Perfectly Poached Eggs.

5. Evenly divide the hash and eggs into microwaveable airtight containers. Reheat in the microwave on high for 1 to 2 minutes, until heated throughout.

SUBSTITUTION TIP: If you're short on time, make scrambled, over easy, or sunny-side-up eggs in a frying pan versus the Perfectly Poached Eggs (page 210).

COOKING TIP: Adding a bit of an acidic ingredient, like vinegar or citrus juice, can mimic the taste of salt in a recipe. We added balsamic vinegar to the vegetables and cut down on the salt while not sacrificing flavor.

VARIATION TIP: Try replacing the sweet potatoes, parsnips, or red onion with a combination of butternut squash, turnips, rutabaga, carrots, or beets.

PER SERVING: Total Calories: 343; Total Fat: 17g; Saturated Fat: 4g; Cholesterol: 422mg; Sodium: 306mg; Potassium: 602mg; Total Carbohydrate: 33g; Fiber: 5g; Sugars: 8g; Protein: 15g

Hash Brown Vegetable Breakfast Casserole

SERVES 6   PREP TIME: 25 MINUTES   COOK TIME: 45 MINUTES

A breakfast casserole is quite possibly the easiest and most delicious way to feed a crowd. It's also perfect for a make-ahead breakfast that can be reheated in the microwave during the week. This version has Greek yogurt for an added boost of protein and probiotics.

12 large eggs

1½ cups plain nonfat Greek yogurt

1 teaspoon onion powder

1 teaspoon garlic powder

½ teaspoon kosher or sea salt

½ teaspoon ground black pepper

¼ teaspoon crushed red pepper flakes

3 cups shredded hash brown potatoes

2 cups baby spinach leaves, roughly chopped

1 red bell pepper, seeded and diced

1½ cups shredded sharp Cheddar cheese, divided

1. Preheat the oven to 375°F. Coat a 9-by-13-inch baking dish with cooking spray.

2. In a large mixing bowl, whisk together the eggs, Greek yogurt, onion powder, garlic powder, salt, black pepper, and red pepper flakes until beaten and combined. Fold in the potatoes, spinach, and red bell pepper and half the sharp Cheddar cheese. Pour the mixture into the prepared baking dish. Sprinkle the remaining shredded cheese evenly over the top.

3. Bake for 35 to 45 minutes, until the egg is set. Remove and allow to slightly cool, then slice into 6 pieces.

4. Store the casserole slices in microwaveable airtight containers and refrigerate for up to 5 days. Reheat by microwaving on high for 60 to 90 seconds, until heated through.

SUBSTITUTION TIP: Try pepper Jack cheese instead of Cheddar for a spicy kick.

COOKING TIP: Make mini versions of this casserole by baking in a muffin tin.

VARIATION TIP: Shredded frozen sweet potatoes can be used instead of regular potatoes for a boost of vitamin A.

PER SERVING: Total Calories: 363; Total Fat: 19g; Saturated Fat: 9g; Cholesterol: 454mg; Sodium: 568mg; Potassium: 169mg; Total Carbohydrate: 21g; Fiber: 3g; Sugars: 2g; Protein: 26g

Sweet Potato Pancakes with Maple Yogurt

SERVES 6 (2 PANCAKES EACH)   PREP TIME: 15 MINUTES   COOK TIME: 20 MINUTES

An easy way to get more vitamin A–packed sweet potatoes into your diet is by adding them to pancake batter. They're mixed with homemade whole-grain pancake mix, pumpkin pie spice, and vanilla, and they're delicious when topped with the maple-infused yogurt.

2 cups whole-wheat flour or whole-wheat pastry flour

1 tablespoon baking powder

1½ teaspoons pumpkin pie spice

½ teaspoon kosher or sea salt

2 tablespoons dark brown sugar

4 tablespoons canola oil

2 large eggs

1 cup sweet potato purée or cooked mashed sweet potato

1½ cups nonfat milk

1 teaspoon pure vanilla extract

Cooking spray

1½ cups plain nonfat Greek yogurt

½ teaspoon maple extract or 1 tablespoon pure maple syrup

1. In a mixing bowl, whisk together the flour, baking powder, pumpkin pie spice, and salt until combined.

2. In a separate mixing bowl, use a hand mixer set on medium speed to beat the brown sugar and canola oil together until fluffy. While the hand mixer is still beating, add one egg at a time until thoroughly combined. Add the sweet potato purée then the milk and vanilla extract until well blended. Turn the hand mixer to low speed and slowly add the dry ingredient mixture until well blended.

3. Heat a large nonstick skillet over medium heat. Coat the pan with the cooking spray. Working in batches, ladle ¼-cup dollops of pancake batter into the pan. Cook for 1 to 2 minutes, until bubbles appear on the top, then flip and cook for another 1 to 2 minutes, until set. Repeat with the remaining batter.

4. In a small bowl, whisk together the Greek yogurt and maple extract or maple syrup until combined. Serve it over the sweet potato pancakes.

5. Store the pancakes in the refrigerator in an airtight container or sealed plastic bag for up to 5 days. Serve chilled or reheat in the microwave on high for 30 seconds. Store the maple yogurt in an airtight container for up to 5 days.

SUBSTITUTION TIP: Gluten-free all-purpose flour can be substituted for regular flour to make this recipe gluten free.

COOKING TIP: How to cook the sweet potatoes: Preheat the oven to 400°F. Poke the potatoes a few times with a fork, then roast them for about an hour, until fork tender. Let them cool, peel, and mash.

VARIATION TIP: Pumpkin purée can be used in place of the mashed sweet potato.

MAKE IT A MEAL: This recipe can be served with lower-sodium chicken sausages or bacon for a higher-protein meal.

PER SERVING: Total Calories: 355; Total Fat: 12g; Saturated Fat: 2g; Cholesterol: 74mg; Sodium: 305mg; Potassium: 477mg; Total Carbohydrate: 50g; Fiber: 6g; Sugars: 14g; Protein: 16g

Whole-Grain Flax Waffles with Strawberry Purée

VEGETARIAN · UNDER 30 MINUTES

SERVES 6   PREP TIME: 15 MINUTES   COOK TIME: 15 MINUTES

Waffles are known for their crisp exterior and fluffy, tender inside, and this version is no exception. We've added a boost of nutrition with whole-wheat pastry flour and flaxseed, but the texture is delicate and mouthwatering. The strawberry purée is a lower-sugar syrup substitute, yet it provides a tangy sweetness that goes perfectly with the waffles.

1 quart strawberries, hulled and chopped

1 cup water

2 tablespoons honey

2½ teaspoons pure vanilla extract, divided

2¼ cups whole-wheat flour or whole-wheat pastry flour

¼ cup ground flaxseed

2½ teaspoons baking powder

1 teaspoon baking soda

½ teaspoon kosher or sea salt

2 teaspoons ground cinnamon

2 tablespoons dark brown sugar

¼ cup canola oil

3 large eggs

1 cup nonfat milk

Cooking spray

1. First, make the strawberry purée: Place the strawberries, water, and honey and ½ teaspoon of vanilla extract in a medium saucepan. Bring to a simmer for 5 to 6 minutes, until the strawberries are soft. Use an immersion blender to purée the strawberries or transfer mixture to a blender and purée until smooth.

2. To make the waffles: In a medium mixing bowl, whisk together the flour, flaxseed, baking powder, baking soda, and salt until combined.

3. In a large mixing bowl, whisk together the ground cinnamon, brown sugar, and canola oil until well combined. Whisk in one egg at a time until the mixture is fluffy. Add the remaining vanilla extract and milk until combined. Slowly whisk the dry ingredients into the wet mixture.

4. Heat a Belgian waffle maker over medium heat. Once hot, coat with the cooking spray. Evenly spoon ⅔ cup batter into the waffle maker. Shut the lid and cook for 1½ to 2 minutes, until the waffle is browned on the outside. Repeat with the remaining batter.

5. Serve the waffles with the strawberry purée.

6. Store the waffles in the refrigerator in an airtight container or sealed plastic bag for up to 5 days. Serve chilled or reheat in the microwave on high for 30 seconds. Store the strawberry purée in an airtight container for up to 5 days.

SUBSTITUTION TIP: We recommend gluten-free all-purpose flour as a celiac-friendly substitution in this recipe. Try oat flour for a higher-fiber gluten-free version of these waffles.

COOKING TIP: To make the waffle batter into pancake batter, reduce the canola oil to 2 tablespoons (instead of ¼ cup), then cook in a greased nonstick skillet set at medium heat for 1 to 2 minutes per side, until set.

VARIATION TIP: Use raspberries or blueberries instead of the strawberries to make the fruit purée.

MAKE IT A MEAL: This recipe can be served with lower-sodium chicken sausages or bacon for a higher-protein meal.

PER SERVING: Total Calories: 381; Total Fat: 15g; Saturated Fat: 2g; Cholesterol: 106mg; Sodium: 459mg; Potassium: 452mg; Total Carbohydrate: 55g; Fiber: 9g; Sugars: 17g; Protein: 12g

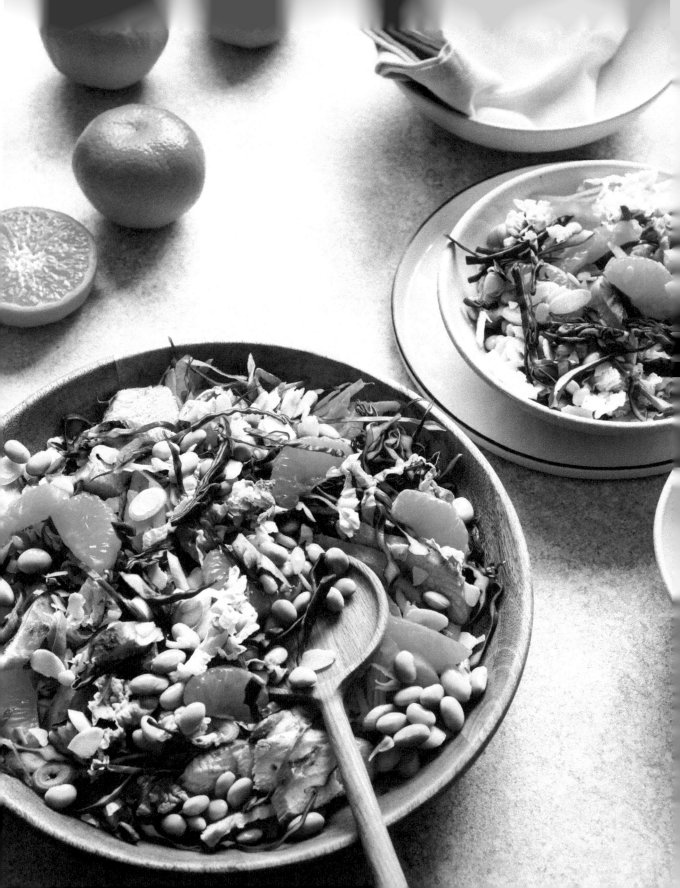

6

Salads, Soups, and Sandwiches

Chicken & Mandarin Orange Salad with Sesame Ginger Dressing

SERVES 4   PREP TIME: 20 MINUTES   COOK TIME: 12 MINUTES

This salad hits all the right notes: It's sweet, savory, crunchy, and a bit nutty. Unlike many salads, this one is a meal-in-one and can be prepped ahead of time. The dressing is loaded with flavor but not salt, unlike many bottled dressings.

FOR THE DRESSING:

¼ cup sodium-free rice wine vinegar

1 tablespoon sesame oil

1 tablespoon honey

2 garlic cloves, peeled and minced

1-inch piece fresh ginger, peeled and minced

¼ teaspoon kosher or sea salt

FOR THE SALAD:

1 tablespoon canola oil

1 pound boneless skinless chicken breasts

¼ teaspoon kosher or sea salt

¼ teaspoon ground black pepper

1 large head Napa cabbage, shredded

1 cup shredded red cabbage

½ cup shredded carrots

½ cup shelled edamame

½ cup sliced almonds

2 scallions, thinly sliced

8-ounce can mandarin oranges, drained

TO MAKE THE DRESSING:

Combine all the dressing ingredients in a jar or bowl and shake or whisk to combine. Refrigerate until ready to use.

TO MAKE THE SALAD:

1. Heat the canola oil in a skillet over medium heat. Season the chicken breasts with the salt and black pepper and place in the skillet. Cook for 5 to 6 minutes per side, until the internal temperature reaches 165°F. Place on a cutting board for 5 to 10 minutes to cool and then thinly slice against the grain.

2. In a large bowl, toss the Napa cabbage, red cabbage, carrots, and edamame together with the dressing. Divide into 4 bowls and top with the sliced chicken, almonds, scallions, and mandarin oranges.

SUBSTITUTION TIP: Use white vinegar if you don't have rice wine vinegar on hand.

COOKING TIP: Prep the dressing and salad ingredients ahead of time and toss together just before lunch or dinner for a simple weekday meal.

VARIATION TIP: Use spinach instead of Napa cabbage if desired.

PER SERVING: Total Calories: 394; Total Fat: 19g; Saturated Fat: 2g; Cholesterol: 70mg; Sodium: 544mg; Potassium: 494mg; Total Carbohydrate: 29g; Fiber: 5g; Sugars: 16g; Protein: 32g

Salmon & Avocado Cobb Salad with Buttermilk Ranch Dressing

SERVES 4   PREP TIME: 20 MINUTES   COOK TIME: 12 MINUTES

The classic Cobb salad gets a DASH-friendly upgrade with fresh salmon and homemade buttermilk ranch dressing. Salmon provides omega-3 fatty acids that are essential for heart and brain health, and our creamy dressing is lower in fat, with loads of fresh herbs and lemon.

FOR THE SALAD:

1 pound salmon fillets, skin removed

1 tablespoon olive oil

¼ teaspoon kosher or sea salt

¼ teaspoon ground black pepper

6 cups romaine lettuce, chopped

1 pint cherry tomatoes, halved

2 large hard-boiled eggs, peeled and quartered

1 avocado, peeled and diced

2 scallions, thinly sliced

FOR THE DRESSING:

⅓ cup low-fat buttermilk

2 tablespoons plain nonfat Greek yogurt

2 tablespoons mayonnaise

Zest and juice of ½ lemon

1 tablespoon chopped fresh herbs of your choice like dill, parsley, or chives

1 to 2 garlic cloves, peeled and minced

½ teaspoon hot sauce

½ teaspoon ground black pepper

¼ teaspoon kosher or sea salt

TO MAKE THE SALAD:

1. Preheat the oven to 400°F. Place the salmon fillets in a greased baking dish. Drizzle with olive oil and season with salt and black pepper. Roast for 8 to 12 minutes, until the salmon flakes easily with a fork. Let slightly cool.

2. Assemble four salads by evenly distributing the romaine, cherry tomatoes, hard-boiled eggs, avocados, and scallions onto 4 large plates or in 4 large containers.

3. Whisk the dressing ingredients until combined.

4. Add the dressing to the salad and toss if serving immediately. Top with the salmon fillet. If storing, keep the salmon fillets and salad in airtight containers for up to 3 days. Store the dressing separately in small airtight containers.

SUBSTITUTION TIP: Use chicken breast, turkey breast, or canned tuna instead of salmon, if desired.

COOKING TIP: Store fresh herbs in a large sealed plastic bag with a paper towel to keep them fresher for longer.

VARIATION TIP: Use spinach instead of romaine lettuce, if desired.

PER SERVING: Total Calories: 365; Total Fat: 23g; Saturated Fat: 4g; Cholesterol: 158mg; Sodium: 486mg; Potassium: 548mg; Total Carbohydrate: 11g; Fiber: 6g; Sugars: 4g; Protein: 30g

Waldorf Chicken Salad

MEAL-IN-ONE

SERVES 4   PREP TIME: 20 MINUTES   COOK TIME: 12 MINUTES

This version of the classic chicken salad has a lightened-up dressing that is full of honey mustard flavor. It's easy to get in the recommended servings of fruits and vegetables when this salad provides at least 4 cups of them! Prep this salad in advance for a quick and easy lunch on the go.

¼ cup plain nonfat Greek yogurt

2 tablespoons mayonnaise

2 tablespoons Dijon mustard

1 tablespoon honey

¼ teaspoon kosher or sea salt

¼ teaspoon ground black pepper

3 cups chopped cooked
   chicken breast

1 apple, diced

2 celery stalks, diced

1 cup green or red seedless
   grapes, halved

¼ cup chopped walnuts

1. In a bowl, whisk together the yogurt, mayonnaise, Dijon mustard, honey, salt, and black pepper. Fold in the cooked chicken, apple, celery, grapes, and walnuts.

2. Store in airtight containers in the refrigerator for up to 3 days.

SUBSTITUTION TIP: Replace chicken with garbanzo beans for a vegetarian version.

COOKING TIP: Be sure to cook the chicken in advance. It can be sautéed in a hot, oiled skillet on the stove or roasted in the oven. Be sure the chicken reaches 165°F, then allow it to fully cool before adding it to the salad.

VARIATION TIP: Use almonds instead of walnuts, if desired.

MAKE IT A MEAL: Serve on whole-wheat bread or with whole-grain crackers.

PER SERVING: Total Calories: 353; Total Fat: 14g; Saturated Fat: 2g; Cholesterol: 92mg; Sodium: 475mg; Potassium: 283mg; Total Carbohydrate: 20g; Fiber: 2g; Sugars: 17g; Protein: 36g

Mediterranean Chickpea Tuna Salad

SERVES 4   PREP TIME: 20 MINUTES

Nothing beats a meal that comes together in minutes without using the oven, stove, or grill. This salad recipe has no lettuce, but it boasts chickpeas, tuna, fresh veggies, feta cheese, and a light lemon oregano dressing, all of which can be prepped ahead for a delicious salad.

FOR THE DRESSING:

2 tablespoons red wine vinegar

Zest and juice of ½ lemon

1 tablespoon honey

1 teaspoon dried oregano leaves

¼ teaspoon kosher or sea salt

¼ teaspoon ground black pepper

¼ cup olive oil

FOR THE SALAD:

1 (15-ounce) can no-salt-added chickpeas, rinsed and drained

1 6.4-ounce pouch albacore tuna

½ English cucumber, diced

1 pint cherry tomatoes, quartered

¼ cup pitted kalamata olives

2 tablespoons crumbled feta cheese

TO MAKE THE DRESSING:

In a bowl, whisk together red wine vinegar, lemon zest and juice, honey, dried oregano, salt, and black pepper. Slowly whisk in the olive oil until combined.

TO MAKE THE SALAD:

1. In a separate bowl, add the chickpeas, tuna, cucumber, tomatoes, olives, and feta cheese.

2. If eating immediately, combine the salad and dressing in a large bowl. If eating later, store the salad and dressing separately in airtight containers. It will stay fresh in the refrigerator for up to 3 days.

COOKING TIP: You can also turn this recipe into Mason jar salads. Evenly distribute the dressing into 4 pint jars. Layer the salad ingredients into each jar, following the order of the ingredients. Shake the salad just before eating to combine the ingredients.

VARIATION TIP: Replace olives with artichokes or roasted red peppers.

MAKE IT A MEAL: Serve with a side of fruit or a handful of whole-grain crackers.

PER SERVING: Total Calories: 347; Total Fat: 20g; Saturated Fat: 2g; Cholesterol: 22mg; Sodium: 574mg; Potassium: 367mg; Total Carbohydrate: 28g; Fiber: 6g; Sugars: 8g; Protein: 17g

Rustic Tomato Panzanella Salad

SERVES 4   PREP TIME: 15 MINUTES   COOK TIME: 8 MINUTES

This traditional Italian salad may have only a few ingredients, but it's the quintessential recipe that contains the highest-quality ingredients prepared in simple ways to really let them shine. If you can, choose heirloom tomatoes at their peak of freshness.

1 small baguette, cubed (about 5 ounces total)

3 tablespoons olive oil, divided

2 to 3 large ripe tomatoes, cubed

1 tablespoon red wine vinegar

¼ teaspoon kosher or sea salt

¼ teaspoon ground black pepper

¼ cup fresh basil leaves, torn

1. Preheat the oven to 400°F.

2. Place the cubed baguette on a baking sheet and drizzle with half of the olive oil. Roast in the oven for 8 minutes, until crisp. Transfer the croutons to a mixing bowl.

3. To the bowl, add the tomatoes, red wine vinegar, salt, black pepper, and remaining olive oil. Toss to combine, and top with the fresh basil. Serve immediately.

SUBSTITUTION TIP: Use balsamic vinegar instead of red wine, if desired.

COOKING TIP: Prep and roast the croutons in advance. Store them in a sealed plastic bag.

VARIATION TIP: Add sliced cucumbers and red onion for a boost of veggies.

MAKE IT A MEAL: Serve with a bowl of soup or half a sandwich.

PER SERVING: Total Calories: 200; Total Fat: 11g; Saturated Fat: 1g; Cholesterol: 0mg; Sodium: 339mg; Potassium: 217mg; Total Carbohydrate: 18g; Fiber: 2g; Sugars: 0g; Protein: 3g

Avocado Egg Salad

VEGETARIAN · UNDER 30 MINUTES

SERVES 4   PREP TIME: 10 MINUTES   COOK TIME: 20 MINUTES

This egg salad boasts heart-healthy monounsaturated fats from the creamy avocado. While it is much lower in saturated fat than typical egg salad, the lemon and herbs provide a light, fresh flavor that you're sure to love. Cook the hard-boiled eggs in advance to make meal prep easy and quick during the week.

8 large eggs

2 avocados, peeled

Zest and juice of ½ lemon

¼ cup flat-leaf Italian parsley, chopped

¼ teaspoon kosher or sea salt

¼ teaspoon ground black pepper

1. Place the eggs in a saucepan and cover with cold water. Bring to a boil, shut the heat off, and place a fitted lid on the top. Set a timer for 17 to 18 minutes. Drain the hot water, and pour cold water over the eggs until cooled. Remove the shells and discard. Cut the eggs into smaller pieces.

2. In a bowl, mash the avocados. Add the eggs to the bowl, along with the lemon zest and juice, Italian parsley, salt, and ground black pepper. Stir to combine and serve.

SUBSTITUTION TIP: Add a tablespoon of mayonnaise to the egg salad for a bit more creaminess, or leave it out for a lower saturated fat option.

COOKING TIP: Avoid using fresh eggs when hard-boiling, as they're more difficult to peel. Use eggs that have been in your refrigerator for at least a week.

VARIATION TIP: For a unique twist, replace lemon and parsley with lime and cilantro.

MAKE IT A MEAL: Serve on whole-wheat bread or with whole-grain crackers, and a side of fruit or veggies.

PER SERVING: Total Calories: 289; Total Fat: 23g; Saturated Fat: 6g; Cholesterol: 422mg; Sodium: 292mg; Potassium: 453mg; Total Carbohydrate: 8g; Fiber: 6g; Sugars: 0g; Protein: 14g

Strawberry, Chicken & Mozzarella Bow Tie Pasta Salad

SERVES 6   PREP TIME: 10 MINUTES   COOK TIME: 20 MINUTES

Making your own salad dressing is as simple as whisking together vinegar or citrus juice, oil, and seasonings. You can also add a bit of mustard, honey, or sugar to balance flavors. When this salad is tossed with whole-grain pasta, fruits, greens, fresh mozzarella, and chicken, it becomes a light yet complete meal.

FOR THE DRESSING:

2 tablespoons balsamic vinegar

1 tablespoon Dijon mustard

1 tablespoon honey

¼ cup olive oil

¼ teaspoon kosher or sea salt

¼ teaspoon ground black pepper

FOR THE SALAD:

8 ounces whole-grain bow tie pasta

1 tablespoon canola oil

½ pound boneless skinless chicken breasts

¼ teaspoon kosher or sea salt

¼ teaspoon ground black pepper

1 quart strawberries, hulled and sliced

1 cup fresh baby spinach

½ cup mini fresh mozzarella balls

¼ cup sliced almonds

FOR THE DRESSING:

In a large bowl, whisk together the dressing ingredients until combined. Taste and adjust seasoning, if necessary.

FOR THE SALAD:

1. Bring a large pot of water to a boil. Cook the pasta according to the package directions.

2. In that same pot, heat the canola oil over medium heat. Season the chicken breasts with the salt and black pepper. Sauté the chicken for 6 to 7 minutes per side, until the internal temperature reaches 165°F. Place on a plate or cutting board to cool. Chop into bite-size pieces.

3. Place the strawberries, spinach, mozzarella, cooled pasta, and diced chicken into the bowl with the dressing and toss to combine. Refrigerate until chilled, and sprinkle the almonds on top before serving.

SUBSTITUTION TIP: To make this vegetarian, skip the chicken breast and serve it as a side dish.

COOKING TIP: When cooking cuts of meat like chicken breast, let them rest after cooking for 5 to 10 minutes before slicing. This helps the meat stay juicy and tender.

VARIATION TIP: Try couscous instead of bow tie pasta.

MAKE IT A MEAL: Serve with sautéed or grilled vegetables.

PER SERVING: Total Calories: 384; Total Fat: 18g; Saturated Fat: 3g; Cholesterol: 33mg; Sodium: 406mg; Potassium: 207mg; Total Carbohydrate: 40g; Fiber: 6g; Sugars: 8g; Protein: 17g

Tuscan Chicken & Kale Soup

MEAL-IN-ONE · UNDER 30 MINUTES

SERVES 6   PREP TIME: 10 MINUTES   COOK TIME: 15 MINUTES

A soup made in under 30 minutes with minimal prep is ideal for busy weeknights. This soup can also be made in advance and eaten throughout the week with a sandwich or salad, or a larger bowl can serve as a complete meal. Don't forget to serve it with a slice of whole-grain baguette.

2 tablespoons olive oil

1 yellow onion, peeled and diced

2 carrots, peeled and diced

2 celery stalks, diced

1 pound boneless skinless chicken breast, cubed

4 cups chopped kale

2 to 3 garlic cloves, peeled and minced

2 tablespoons dried Italian seasoning

½ teaspoon kosher or sea salt

½ teaspoon ground black pepper

1 (15-ounce) can cannellini beans, rinsed and drained

1 (15-ounce) can no-salt-added petite diced tomatoes with juice

4 cups unsalted chicken stock

½ cup freshly grated Parmesan cheese

1. In a Dutch oven or stockpot, heat the oil over medium heat. Add the onion, carrots, and celery and cook for 3 to 4 minutes, until they start to soften. Stir in the cubed chicken breast and cook for 3 to 4 minutes, until slightly browned on the edges. Stir in the kale, garlic, Italian seasoning, salt, and black pepper until the kale is slightly wilted.

2. Add the cannellini beans, diced tomatoes, and stock and bring to a simmer for about 10 minutes, stirring occasionally. Taste and adjust the seasoning, if necessary.

3. Divide the soup evenly into bowls and top with the grated Parmesan.

4. Divide leftovers evenly into microwaveable airtight containers and store in the refrigerator for up to 5 days. Reheat in the microwave on high for 2 to 3 minutes, until heated through, stirring as needed.

SUBSTITUTION TIP: To make this vegetarian, skip the chicken breast and add another can of cannellini beans.

COOKING TIP: To make in the slow cooker: Place ingredient-list amounts of onion, carrots, celery, chicken breast, kale, garlic, Italian seasoning, salt, black pepper, cannellini beans, diced tomatoes with juice, and chicken stock in the bowl of a slow cooker. Cook on low for 7 to 8 hours or high for 3 to 4 hours.

VARIATION TIP: Try lower-sodium ground Italian turkey sausage instead of chicken.

PER SERVING: Total Calories: 267; Total Fat: 9g; Saturated Fat: 3g; Cholesterol: 53mg; Sodium: 543mg; Potassium: 195mg; Total Carbohydrate: 23g; Fiber: 6g; Sugars: 5g; Protein: 24g

Cauliflower Leek Soup

VEGETARIAN

SERVES 6   PREP TIME: 15 MINUTES   COOK TIME: 25 MINUTES

This soup is so easy to make, yet your friends and family will think it's restaurant-quality because of its luxurious puréed texture and perfectly balanced flavors.

1 tablespoon canola oil

1 yellow onion, peeled and diced

1 leek, trimmed and thinly sliced

1 head cauliflower, trimmed and cut into florets

2 to 3 garlic cloves, peeled and minced

2 tablespoons fresh thyme leaves, chopped

1¼ teaspoons kosher or sea salt

1 teaspoon smoked paprika

½ teaspoon ground black pepper

¼ teaspoon ground cayenne pepper

3 cups unsalted vegetable stock

1 tablespoon heavy cream or olive oil

Zest and juice of ½ lemon

1. Heat the canola oil in a Dutch oven or stockpot over medium heat. Add the onion, leek, and cauliflower and sauté for 4 to 5 minutes, until the onion is starting to soften. Stir in the garlic, thyme, salt, smoked paprika, black pepper, and cayenne pepper. Add the vegetable stock and bring to a simmer for about 15 minutes, until the cauliflower is very soft.

2. Remove from the heat and stir in the cream or olive oil and lemon zest and juice. Use an immersion blender to purée the soup until smooth, or transfer the soup to a blender and purée in batches until smooth. Taste and adjust the seasoning, if necessary.

3. If you are not eating the soup right away, transfer it into microwaveable airtight containers and refrigerate for up to 5 days. Reheat in the microwave on high for 1 to 3 minutes, until heated through.

SUBSTITUTION TIP: Use olive oil or heavy cream to finish the soup for a luxurious richness. Olive oil has mostly monounsaturated fats whereas heavy cream has mostly saturated fats, but when using it in small amounts, you're still able to achieve your nutrition goals.

COOKING TIP: Adding a bit of an acidic ingredient, like vinegar or citrus juice, can mimic the taste of salt in a recipe. We added lemon juice to this soup to cut down the salt while not sacrificing flavor.

VARIATION TIP: Replace lemon zest and juice with balsamic vinegar for a unique flavor.

MAKE IT A MEAL: Serve with half a sandwich to make it a meal.

PER SERVING: Total Calories: 92; Total Fat: 4g; Saturated Fat: 1g; Cholesterol: 3mg; Sodium: 556mg; Potassium: 526mg; Total Carbohydrate: 13g; Fiber: 4g; Sugars: 4g; Protein: 5g

White Bean, Chicken & Green Chili

MEAL-IN-ONE

SERVES 6   PREP TIME: 20 MINUTES   COOK TIME: 25 MINUTES

Tomatillos, generally known as husk tomatoes, are traditionally used to make salsa verde. They look like green tomatoes and have a crisp shell on their exterior, which is peeled before the tomatillos are cooked or consumed. They may seem intimidating, but they're mild in flavor and are packed with essential vitamins and minerals.

2 pounds tomatillos, peeled and quartered

1 jalapeño, halved and seeded

½ red onion, peeled

2 tablespoons canola oil, divided

1½ cups unsalted chicken stock

3 (15-ounce) cans great northern beans, rinsed and drained, divided

1 tablespoon ground cumin

½ teaspoon coarse salt

½ teaspoon ground black pepper

1 pound boneless skinless chicken breast, cubed

2 (4-ounce) cans green chiles with juice

½ cup fresh cilantro leaves, chopped

Zest and juice of 1 lime

Pinch granulated sugar (optional)

¼ cup plain nonfat Greek yogurt

1. Preheat the oven to 425°F.

2. Place the tomatillos, jalapeño, and red onion on a baking sheet and toss with 1 tablespoon of the canola oil. Roast for 20 minutes, until the vegetables are caramelized on the edges.

3. Transfer the caramelized vegetables to a blender or food processor. Add the chicken stock, 1 (15-ounce) can of beans, cumin, salt, and black pepper to the blender or food processor. Purée until smooth.

4. In a Dutch oven or stockpot, heat the remaining 1 tablespoon canola oil over medium heat. Add the cubed chicken breast and sauté for 4 to 5 minutes, until fully cooked. Add the remaining two cans of beans, green chiles, chopped cilantro, lime zest and juice, and puréed mixture to the pot and simmer for about 10 minutes. Taste the soup, and if tart, add the pinch of granulated sugar.

5. Evenly divide the soup into bowls and garnish with the Greek yogurt.

6. Divide leftovers evenly into microwaveable airtight containers and store in the refrigerator for up to 5 days. Reheat in the microwave on high for 2 to 3 minutes, until heated through, stirring as needed.

SUBSTITUTION TIP: To make this vegetarian, skip the chicken breast and add another can of great northern beans.

COOKING TIP: Roasting the vegetables before adding them to the soup imparts a greater depth of flavor from the caramelization process.

VARIATION TIP: Try cutting down on the amount of stock to make a thicker stew and serve it over brown rice.

MAKE IT A MEAL: This chili can be paired with half a sandwich or a salad.

PER SERVING: Total Calories: 356; Total Fat:8 g; Saturated Fat: 1g; Cholesterol: 47mg; Sodium: 566mg; Potassium: 460mg; Total Carbohydrate: 42g; Fiber: 12g; Sugars: 9g; Protein: 29g

Shrimp & Corn Chowder

MEAL-IN-ONE

SERVES 6   PREP TIME: 20 MINUTES   COOK TIME: 30 MINUTES

This Southern-style soup is low in fat and sodium but loaded with flavor. It boasts large pieces of shrimp, corn, and potatoes with a deliciously creamy broth. When made in advance, it can be quickly heated up for a cozy, savory meal on a busy day.

3 tablespoons canola oil

1 yellow onion, peeled and diced

2 carrots, peeled and sliced

2 celery stalks, diced

4 baby Yukon Gold or red potatoes, diced

3 to 4 garlic cloves, peeled and minced

¼ cup all-purpose flour

3 cups unsalted vegetable or chicken stock

½ cup milk

¾ teaspoon kosher or sea salt

¼ teaspoon ground black pepper

¼ teaspoon ground cayenne pepper

4 cups fresh or frozen corn kernels

1 pound raw shrimp, peeled, deveined, and tails removed, chopped

2 scallions, thinly sliced

1. In a Dutch oven or stockpot, heat the oil over medium heat. Add the onion, carrots, celery, and potatoes to the pot. Cook for 5 to 7 minutes, until the vegetables are softened. Stir in the garlic and soften for one minute. Then stir in the flour to make a roux. Increase the heat to medium-high and slowly whisk in the stock and bring to a simmer, taking care to whisk out any lumps of roux so the stock is smooth. After the roux starts to turn brown, whisk in the milk, salt, black pepper, and cayenne pepper. Let simmer, stirring regularly, until thickened, 7 to 8 minutes.

2. Add the corn and shrimp and simmer for an additional 4 to 5 minutes, until the shrimp is fully cooked. Taste and adjust the seasoning, if necessary.

3. Divide the soup evenly into bowls and top with sliced scallions.

4. For leftovers, divide the chowder evenly into microwaveable airtight containers and store in the refrigerator for up to 5 days. Reheat in the microwave on high for 2 to 3 minutes, until heated through, stirring as needed.

SUBSTITUTION TIP: If using fresh corn, carefully slice the corn kernels off the cob. Five or six medium cobs will yield about 4 cups kernels.

COOKING TIP: To make in the slow cooker: Place the onion, carrots, celery, potatoes, garlic, stock, milk, salt, black pepper, cayenne pepper, and corn in the bowl of a slow cooker. Cook on low for 7 to 8 hours or high for 3 to 4 hours. In a small bowl, whisk together 3 tablespoons cornstarch with 1 tablespoon water. Pour the mixture into the slow cooker along with the shrimp and cook an additional 30 minutes on high.

VARIATION TIP: Use chicken breast instead of shrimp, if desired.

PER SERVING: Total Calories: 340; Total Fat: 9g; Saturated Fat: 1g; Cholesterol: 115mg; Sodium: 473mg; Potassium: 613mg; Total Carbohydrate: 45g; Fiber: 5g; Sugars: 8g; Protein: 23g

Classic Beef & Bean Chili

MEAL-IN-ONE

SERVES 8   PREP TIME: 15 MINUTES   COOK TIME: 25 MINUTES

Chili is the perfect make-ahead meal for the colder months. Soups, chili, and casseroles actually gain flavor as they sit because the ingredients have a chance to meld. Plus, the topping options are endless, making chili night a fun experience for the whole family.

1 tablespoon canola oil

1 yellow onion, peeled and diced

1½ pounds lean ground beef

5 to 6 garlic cloves, peeled and minced

3 tablespoons chili powder

1 teaspoon kosher or sea salt

½ teaspoon ground black pepper

2 tablespoons no-salt-added tomato paste

1 (32-ounce) can no-salt-added crushed tomatoes

2 (15-ounce) cans no-salt-added dark red kidney beans, rinsed and drained

2 cups unsalted beef stock

2 avocados, peeled and diced

½ cup shredded sharp Cheddar cheese

1. Heat the oil in a Dutch oven or stockpot over medium heat. Add the onion and sauté for 3 to 4 minutes, until the onion is starting to soften. Add the ground beef and cook, breaking it up into smaller pieces, until the beef is browned. Stir in the garlic, chili powder, salt, black pepper, and tomato paste and cook for 1 minute.

2. Add the crushed tomatoes, kidney beans, and beef stock and bring to a simmer. Cook for 15 minutes. Taste and adjust the seasoning, if necessary.

3. Divide the chili evenly into bowls and top with the diced avocados and shredded Cheddar cheese.

4. Transfer leftover chili into microwaveable airtight containers, top with shredded Cheddar cheese, and refrigerate for up to 5 days. Reheat in the microwave on high for 1 to 3 minutes, until heated through, and top with avocado.

VARIATION TIP: Some great add-ins include green chiles, cumin, and fresh cilantro.

PER SERVING: Total Calories: 363; Total Fat: 17g; Saturated Fat: 5g; Cholesterol: 59mg; Sodium: 526mg; Potassium: 344mg; Total Carbohydrate: 29g; Fiber: 10g; Sugars: 6g; Protein: 26g

Spinach & Artichoke Grilled Cheese

VEGETARIAN · UNDER 30 MINUTES

SERVES 4   PREP TIME: 15 MINUTES   COOK TIME: 15 MINUTES

We've lightened up the traditional spinach artichoke dip a bit by using Greek yogurt and loads of spinach. And instead of dipping, our mixture is the filling for a grilled cheese sandwich on crispy whole-wheat bread. Don't be afraid to get your hands messy when eating this one!

2 cups baby spinach leaves, chopped

1 cup jarred marinated artichoke hearts, chopped

¼ cup nonfat plain Greek yogurt

2 to 3 garlic cloves, peeled and minced

¼ teaspoon ground black pepper

⅛ teaspoon kosher or sea salt

8 slices whole-wheat bread

4 slices mozzarella cheese

1 tablespoon olive oil

1. In a bowl, mix together the spinach, artichoke hearts, Greek yogurt, garlic, black pepper, and salt until combined.

2. Heat a skillet to medium. Prepare the sandwiches by placing 4 slices bread on a cutting board. Evenly distribute the spinach artichoke mixture onto each slice and top with a slice of mozzarella cheese. Top with another slice of bread. Brush top slices of bread with the olive oil. Place the sandwiches olive oil-side down in the hot skillet. Cook for 2 to 3 minutes, until browned. Brush the other slices of bread with the olive oil, then flip and cook for another 2 to 3 minutes, until the bottom is browned and the cheese is melted. Place a lid over the skillet, if necessary, to assist with melting the cheese.

3. Slice each sandwich in half and serve.

SUBSTITUTION TIP: To make this gluten free, use gluten-free bread.

COOKING TIP: To achieve a golden, crispy crust on the bread, make sure the skillet is hot before placing the sandwiches in.

VARIATION TIP: Use roasted red peppers instead of artichokes, if desired.

MAKE IT A MEAL: Serve with a side of fruit or vegetables.

PER SERVING: Total Calories: 355; Total Fat: 13g; Saturated Fat: 4g; Cholesterol: 11mg; Sodium: 511mg; Potassium: 53mg; Total Carbohydrate: 44g; Fiber: 9g; Sugars: 7g; Protein: 16g

Chipotle Chicken & Caramelized Onion Panini

SERVES 8   PREP TIME: 20 MINUTES   COOK TIME: 25 MINUTES

A hearty panini with sweet caramelized onions, juicy chicken, and gooey cheese can seem like a sin when trying to reach nutrition goals. But this version boasts loads of potassium, protein, and fiber and is lower in saturated fat and sugar than most meals, so you can feel good about eating something tasty and something DASH-friendly!

2 tablespoons canola oil, divided

2 yellow onions, thinly sliced

½ pound boneless skinless chicken breasts, thinly sliced

2 tablespoons Honey Chipotle Sauce (page 221)

8 slices store-bought whole-wheat bread or Honey Whole-Wheat Bread (page 224)

4 slices low-sodium provolone cheese

1 tablespoon olive oil

1. In a large skillet, heat 2 tablespoons canola oil over medium-low heat. Add the onions and cook for 20 minutes, stirring occasionally, until they are soft and caramel colored on the edges. Place them in a bowl and set aside.

2. In the same skillet, add another tablespoon of canola oil over medium heat. Place the chicken in the skillet and cook for 3 to 4 minutes per side, until the chicken reaches 165°F. Transfer the cooked chicken to the bowl with the caramelized onions and stir in the honey chipotle sauce until combined.

3. Wipe out the skillet and put back on the range. Prepare the sandwiches by placing 4 slices of bread on a cutting board. Evenly distribute the chicken/onion mixture onto each slice and top with a slice of provolone cheese. Top with another slice of bread. Brush the top slices of bread with olive oil. Place the sandwiches olive oil–side down in the hot skillet. Cook for 2 to 3 minutes, until browned. Brush the other slices of bread with olive oil, then flip and cook for another 2 to 3 minutes, until the bottom is browned and the cheese is melted. Place a lid over the skillet, if necessary, to assist with melting the cheese.

4. Slice each sandwich in half and serve.

SUBSTITUTION TIP: If you don't have time to make the sauce, grab a bottle of lower-sodium barbecue sauce instead.

COOKING TIP: Prep or cook the onions, chicken, and Honey Chipotle Sauce (page 221) in advance to make panini-making quick and easy when it's time to eat.

VARIATION TIP: Try Gouda or Havarti cheese instead of provolone.

MAKE IT A MEAL: Serve the paninis with a side of fresh fruit or vegetables to make a complete meal.

PER SERVING: Total Calories: 260; Total Fat: 11g; Saturated Fat: 3g; Cholesterol: 26mg; Sodium: 308mg; Potassium: 67mg; Total Carbohydrate: 25g; Fiber: 3.5g; Sugars: 7g; Protein: 20g

Crispy Fish Sandwiches with Creamy Coleslaw

SERVES 8   PREP TIME: 20 MINUTES   COOK TIME: 10 MINUTES

Instead of going out on a Friday night, opt to make your own crispy fish and coleslaw with just as much flavor and crunch but without the extra fat and calories. This whitefish is breaded and sautéed to perfection, and the coleslaw is creamy and tangy, just like it should be.

FOR THE COLESLAW:

- ¼ cup plain nonfat Greek yogurt
- 2 tablespoons mayonnaise
- 1 tablespoon dried minced onion
- 1 tablespoon granulated sugar
- 1 tablespoon white wine vinegar
- ½ tablespoon dry mustard powder
- ½ tablespoon celery seed
- ¼ teaspoon kosher or sea salt
- ¼ teaspoon ground black pepper
- 4 ounces green cabbage, diced
- 4 ounces carrots, peeled and diced

FOR THE SANDWICHES:

- ⅓ cup all-purpose flour
- 1 large egg, beaten
- 2 tablespoons milk
- ⅔ cup panko bread crumbs
- ¼ teaspoon kosher or sea salt
- ½ teaspoon ground black pepper
- 3 tablespoons canola oil
- 2 pounds whitefish (cod, haddock, tilapia) fillets, cut into 4-ounce pieces
- 8 whole-wheat sandwich buns, toasted

TO MAKE THE COLESLAW:

In a bowl, whisk together the Greek yogurt, mayonnaise, onion, sugar, white wine vinegar, dry mustard, celery seed, salt, and black pepper. Fold in the green cabbage and carrots until combined. Refrigerate until use.

TO MAKE THE SANDWICHES:

1. Set up a breading station: one with the flour, one with the mixed beaten egg and milk, and one with the bread crumbs. Evenly distribute the salt and black pepper into each bowl and whisk each to thoroughly combine.

2. Heat the canola oil in a large skillet over medium heat.

3. Dip each fish fillet in the flour, egg mixture, then bread crumbs and place in the hot oil. Repeat with the remaining fish fillets, working in batches if needed. Cook the fish until all sides are crispy and browned and the fish flakes easily with a fork. Place the fish fillets on the whole-wheat buns and top with the coleslaw.

4. You can prep the crispy fish in advance. For reheating, it is recommended to broil fish in the oven set on low for 2 to 3 minutes per side. The coleslaw should be stored in an airtight container in the refrigerator for up to 3 days.

SUBSTITUTION TIP: To make this recipe gluten free, choose gluten-free panko bread crumbs and gluten-free sandwich buns.

COOKING TIP: Make the coleslaw a few hours or one day in advance to allow the flavors to meld.

VARIATION TIP: Make this recipe into fish sticks or nuggets by cutting them into smaller pieces before breading and sautéing.

MAKE IT A MEAL: Serve with a side of roasted or grilled vegetables.

PER SERVING: Total Calories: 396; Total Fat: 12g; Saturated Fat: 1g; Cholesterol: 28mg; Sodium: 504mg; Potassium: 109mg; Total Carbohydrate: 45g; Fiber: 6g; Sugars: 10g; Protein: 33g

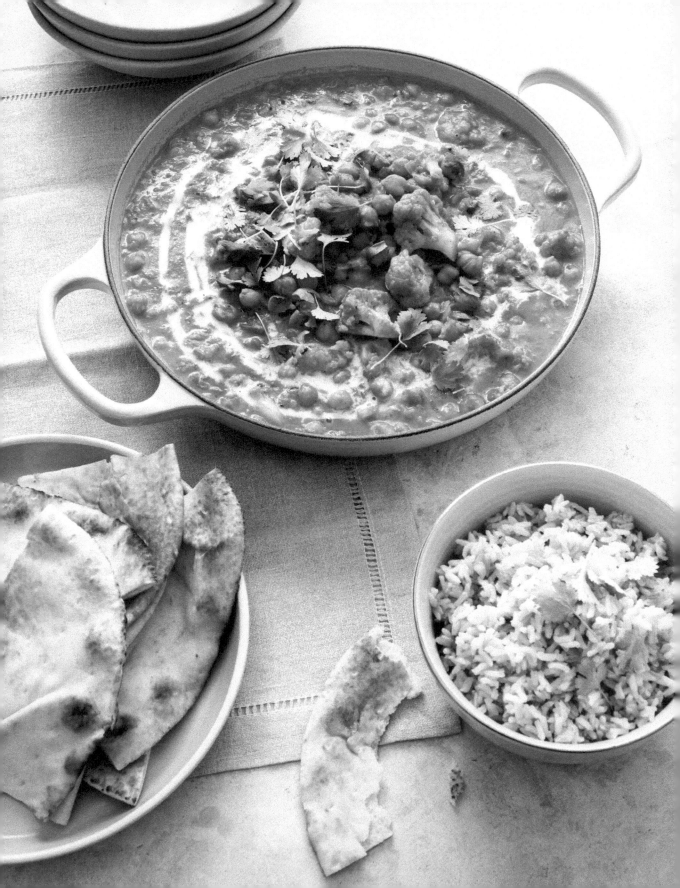

Meatless Mains

Hummus & Vegetable–Stuffed Collard Wraps

VEGAN · MEAL-IN-ONE · UNDER 30 MINUTES

SERVES 6   PREP TIME: 25 MINUTES

Raw collard greens are the vehicle that hold together a rainbow of veggies, creamy avocado, and a smattering of earthy hummus. Not only are these wraps loaded with fiber, they are a great source of several vitamins and minerals.

4 large collard leaves

1 cup Homemade Hummus (page 218) or store-bought hummus

2 avocados, peeled and sliced

1 orange, red, or yellow bell pepper, thinly sliced

½ English cucumber, cut into matchsticks

1 cup shredded red cabbage

1 cup shredded carrots

1 cup alfalfa sprouts

1. Lay collard leaves flat on a cutting board. Spread the hummus in the center of each leaf. Evenly stack the avocado slices, bell pepper slices, cucumber, cabbage, carrot, and alfalfa sprouts on each. Fold the ends in and roll like a burrito. Slice each wrap in half.

2. Store in airtight containers for up to 3 days.

SUBSTITUTION TIP: Choose a lower-sodium hummus by comparing the nutrition facts of similar brands and flavors.

COOKING TIP: Use a paring knife to remove large stalks from the base of the collard wraps to make them easier to roll and to eat.

VARIATION TIP: Try using whole-grain tortillas instead of collard wraps, if desired.

MAKE IT A MEAL: For a higher-protein meat version, add cooked chicken or turkey breast.

PER SERVING: Total Calories: 196; Total Fat: 13g; Saturated Fat: 2g; Cholesterol: 0mg; Sodium: 185mg; Potassium: 531mg; Total Carbohydrate: 18g; Fiber: 9g; Sugars: 2g; Protein: 6g

Tofu & Green Bean Stir-Fry

VEGETARIAN · MEAL-IN-ONE

SERVES 4   PREP TIME: 20 MINUTES   COOK TIME: 20 MINUTES

Stir-fried dishes are perfect for weeknights because the cooking process is quick, especially if the sauce is made in advance. Prep a batch of Fluffy Brown Rice (page 223) on the weekend and use it for meals throughout the week.

1 (14-ounce) package extra-firm tofu

2 tablespoons canola oil

1 pound green beans, chopped

2 carrots, peeled and thinly sliced

½ cup Stir-Fry Sauce (page 222) or store-bought lower-sodium stir-fry sauce

2 cups Fluffy Brown Rice (page 223)

2 scallions, thinly sliced

2 tablespoons sesame seeds

1. Remove the tofu from the package and place it on a plate lined with a kitchen towel. Place another kitchen towel on top of the tofu and place a heavy pot on top, changing towels if they become soaked. Let sit for 15 minutes to remove the moisture. Cut the tofu into 1-inch cubes.

2. Heat the canola oil in a large wok or skillet to medium-high heat. Add the tofu cubes and cook, flipping every 1 to 2 minutes so all sides become browned. Remove from the skillet and place the green beans and carrots in the hot oil. Stir-fry for 4 to 5 minutes, tossing occasionally, until crisp and slightly tender.

3. While the vegetables are cooking, prepare the Stir-Fry Sauce (if using homemade).

4. Place the tofu back in the skillet. Pour the sauce over the tofu and vegetables and let simmer for 2 to 3 minutes.

5. Serve the stir-fry over rice and top with scallions and sesame seeds.

6. For leftovers, divide the stir-fry evenly into microwaveable airtight containers and store in the refrigerator for up to 5 days. Reheat in the microwave on high for 2 to 3 minutes, until heated through.

SUBSTITUTION TIP: Try seitan instead of tofu. It also is a great source of protein and lends itself well to Asian-style dishes.

PER SERVING: Total Calories: 380; Total Fat: 15g; Saturated Fat: 2g; Cholesterol: 0mg; Sodium: 440mg; Potassium: 454mg; Total Carbohydrate: 45g; Fiber: 8g; Sugars: 11g; Protein: 16g

Peanut Vegetable Pad Thai

VEGAN · MEAL-IN-ONE

SERVES 6   PREP TIME: 25 MINUTES   COOK TIME: 20 MINUTES

Pad Thai may seem like an intimidating dish to cook, but most of the prep can be done in advance. Whisk up the sauce and chop the vegetables when you have more time, and take just 20 minutes when you are ready to whip up this classic noodle dish.

8 ounces brown rice noodles

⅓ cup natural peanut butter

3 tablespoons unsalted vegetable broth

1 tablespoon low-sodium soy sauce

2 tablespoons rice wine vinegar

1 tablespoon honey

2 teaspoons sesame oil

1 teaspoon sriracha (optional)

1 tablespoon canola oil

1 red bell pepper, seeded and thinly sliced

1 zucchini, cut into matchsticks

2 large carrots, cut into matchsticks

3 large eggs, beaten

¾ teaspoon kosher or sea salt

½ cup unsalted peanuts, chopped

½ cup cilantro leaves, chopped

1. Bring a large pot of water to a boil. Cook the rice noodles according to package directions.

2. In a bowl, whisk together the peanut butter, vegetable broth, soy sauce, rice wine vinegar, honey, sesame oil, and sriracha (if using) until combined. Set aside.

3. In a large nonstick skillet, heat the canola oil over medium heat. Add the red bell pepper, zucchini, and carrots, and sauté for 2 to 3 minutes, until slightly soft. Stir in the eggs and fold with a spatula until scrambled. Add the cooked rice noodles, sauce, and salt. Toss to combine.

4. Spoon into bowls and evenly top with the peanuts and cilantro.

5. For leftovers, divide into microwaveable airtight containers and store in the refrigerator for up to 5 days. Reheat in the microwave on high for 2 to 3 minutes, until heated through, stirring as needed.

SUBSTITUTION TIP: For a gluten-free version, use low-sodium tamari instead of soy sauce.

VARIATION TIP: If you have a vegetable spiralizer, you can spiralize the red bell pepper, zucchini, and 2 large carrots to create vegetable noodles instead of brown rice noodles.

MAKE IT A MEAL: Serve with a side of fresh fruit.

PER SERVING: Total Calories: 393; Total Fat: 19g; Saturated Fat: 3g; Cholesterol: 105mg; Sodium: 561mg; Potassium: 309mg; Total Carbohydrate: 45g; Fiber: 7g; Sugars: 7g; Protein: 13g

Spicy Tofu Burrito Bowls with Cilantro Avocado Sauce

SERVES 4   PREP TIME: 20 MINUTES   COOK TIME: 15 MINUTES

The cilantro avocado sauce can be made in advance and used throughout the week in many recipes. It adds flavor, moisture, and a boost of protein and heart-healthy fats from the avocado and Greek yogurt. You can also make the burrito bowls in advance and reheat them for lunch during the week.

FOR THE SAUCE:

- ¼ cup plain nonfat Greek yogurt or low-fat sour cream
- ½ cup fresh cilantro leaves
- ½ ripe avocado, peeled
- Zest and juice of 1 lime
- 2 garlic cloves, peeled
- ¼ teaspoon kosher or sea salt
- 2 tablespoons water

FOR THE BURRITO BOWLS:

- 1 (14-ounce) package extra-firm tofu
- 1 tablespoon canola oil
- 1 yellow or orange bell pepper, diced
- 2 tablespoons Taco Seasoning (page 216)
- ¼ teaspoon kosher or sea salt
- 2 cups Fluffy Brown Rice (page 223)
- 1 (15-ounce) can black beans, rinsed and drained

TO MAKE THE SAUCE:

Place all the sauce ingredients in the bowl of a food processor or blender and purée until smooth. Taste and adjust the seasoning, if necessary. Refrigerate until ready for use.

TO MAKE THE BURRITO BOWLS:

1. Remove the tofu from the package and place it on a plate lined with a kitchen towel. Place another kitchen towel on top of the tofu and place a heavy pot on top, changing towels if they become soaked. Let sit for 15 minutes to remove the moisture. Cut the tofu into 1-inch cubes.

2. Heat the canola oil in a large skillet over medium heat. Add the tofu and bell pepper and sauté, breaking up the tofu into smaller pieces, for 4 to 5 minutes, until the peppers are soft. Stir in the taco seasoning, salt, and ¼ cup of water.

3. Evenly divide the rice and black beans among 4 bowls. Top with the tofu/bell pepper mixture and top with the cilantro avocado sauce.

4. For leftovers, divide evenly into microwaveable airtight containers and store in the refrigerator for up to 5 days. Reheat in the microwave on high for 1 to 3 minutes, until heated through.

SUBSTITUTION TIP: For a meat version, try ground chicken, turkey, or beef.

COOKING TIP: This dish works best with extra-firm tofu because it gets a crispy browned exterior when sautéed.

VARIATION TIP: Swap out the tofu with roasted, cubed sweet potatoes.

PER SERVING: Total Calories: 383; Total Fat: 13g; Saturated Fat: 2g; Cholesterol: 1mg; Sodium: 438mg; Potassium: 297mg; Total Carbohydrate: 48g; Fiber: 9g; Sugars: 2g; Protein: 21g

Sweet Potato Cakes with Classic Guacamole

VEGAN • MEAL-IN-ONE

SERVES 4   PREP TIME: 15 MINUTES   COOK TIME: 20 MINUTES

Sweet potatoes and black beans are the base of these vegetarian cakes, with a spicy twist from chili powder and cumin. The guacamole adds heart-healthy monounsaturated fats from avocado and loads of flavor from the jalapeño, red onion, cilantro, and lime. While the sweet potato cakes cook, whip up the guacamole for a quick and easy weeknight meal.

FOR THE GUACAMOLE:

2 ripe avocados, peeled and pitted

½ jalapeño, seeded and finely minced

¼ red onion, peeled and finely diced

¼ cup fresh cilantro leaves, chopped

Zest and juice of 1 lime

¼ teaspoon kosher or sea salt

FOR THE CAKES:

3 sweet potatoes, cooked and peeled

½ cup cooked black beans

1 large egg

½ cup panko bread crumbs

1 teaspoon ground cumin

1 teaspoon chili powder

½ teaspoon kosher or sea salt

¼ teaspoon ground black pepper

2 tablespoons canola oil

TO MAKE THE GUACAMOLE:

In a bowl, mash the avocado, then stir in the jalapeño, red onion, cilantro, lime zest and juice, and salt until combined. Taste and adjust the seasoning, if necessary.

TO MAKE THE CAKES:

1. Place the cooked sweet potatoes and black beans in a bowl and mash until a paste forms. Stir in the egg, bread crumbs, cumin, chili powder, salt, and black pepper until combined.

2. Heat the canola oil in a large skillet at medium heat. Form the sweet potato mixture into 4 patties, place them each in the hot skillet, and cook for 3 to 4 minutes per side, until browned and crispy.

3. Serve the sweet potato cakes with guacamole on top.

SUBSTITUTION TIP: If you don't have sweet potatoes, use an entire 15-ounce can of black beans instead.

COOKING TIP: You can also bake these cakes. Preheat the oven to 400°F, make the cakes, place them on a baking sheet, and roast for 20 minutes, until set and crispy on the outside.

VARIATION TIP: To make these into a party appetizer, make the cakes bite-size and serve with a dollop of guacamole on top.

PER SERVING: Total Calories: 369; Total Fat: 22g; Saturated Fat: 3g; Cholesterol: 53mg; Sodium: 521mg; Potassium: 991mg; Total Carbohydrate: 38g; Fiber: 12g; Sugars: 7g; Protein: 8g

Chickpea Cauliflower Tikka Masala

VEGAN · MEAL-IN-ONE

SERVES 6   PREP TIME: 30 MINUTES   COOK TIME: 40 MINUTES

Garam masala is a spice mixture used in traditional Indian dishes. To make your own, head to page 215, or you can find it in most grocery stores. Most brands have their own unique mix, so one will not necessarily be the same as another.

2 tablespoons olive oil

1 yellow onion, peeled and diced

4 garlic cloves, peeled and minced

1-inch piece fresh ginger, peeled and minced

2 tablespoons Garam Masala (page 215)

1 teaspoon kosher or sea salt

½ teaspoon ground black pepper

¼ teaspoon ground cayenne pepper

½ small head cauliflower, trimmed and cut into small florets (about 2 cups)

2 (15-ounce) cans no-salt-added chickpeas, rinsed and drained

1 (15-ounce) can no-salt-added petite diced tomatoes, drained

1½ cups unsalted vegetable broth

½ (15-ounce) can coconut milk

Zest and juice of 1 lime

½ cup fresh cilantro leaves, chopped, divided

1½ cups cooked Fluffy Brown Rice (page 223), divided

1. In a large Dutch oven or stockpot, heat the olive oil over medium heat. Add the onion and sauté for 4 to 5 minutes, until soft. Stir in the garlic, ginger, garam masala, salt, black pepper, and cayenne pepper and toast for 30 to 60 seconds, until fragrant. Stir in the cauliflower florets, chickpeas, diced tomatoes, and vegetable broth and increase the heat to medium-high. Simmer for 15 minutes, until the cauliflower is fork tender.

2. Remove from the heat and stir in the coconut milk, lime juice, and lime zest and half of the cilantro. Taste and adjust the seasoning, if necessary.

3. Serve over the rice and the remaining chopped cilantro.

4. For leftovers, divide into microwaveable airtight containers and store in the refrigerator for up to 5 days. Reheat in the microwave on high for 2 to 3 minutes, until heated through, stirring as needed.

SUBSTITUTION TIP: Try using cooked quinoa instead of rice for a boost of protein.

COOKING TIP: Before measuring the coconut milk into the pot, thoroughly whisk it to combine the fat and water. Also, you can purchase prechopped cauliflower florets in the produce section to save on prep time.

VARIATION TIP: For a meat version of this dish, replace the cauliflower with one pound of cubed boneless skinless chicken breast.

PER SERVING: Total Calories: 323; Total Fat: 12g; Saturated Fat: 5g; Cholesterol: 0mg; Sodium: 444mg; Potassium: 430mg; Total Carbohydrate: 44g; Fiber: 9g; Sugars: 8g; Protein: 11g

Eggplant Parmesan Stacks

SERVES 4   PREP TIME: 20 MINUTES   COOK TIME: 20 MINUTES

Eggplant Parmesan is a quintessential vegetarian entrée, and for good reason. Eggplant has a hearty, meaty texture and holds up even when smothered with hot marinara and melted fresh mozzarella. Instead of breading the eggplant, we roasted it at a high temperature and layered it with a bread crumb, garlic, and Parmesan cheese mixture, making it quicker and easier to execute.

1 large eggplant, cut into thick slices

2 tablespoons olive oil, divided

¼ teaspoon kosher or sea salt

¼ teaspoon ground black pepper

1 cup panko bread crumbs

¼ cup freshly grated Parmesan cheese

5 to 6 garlic cloves, peeled
   and minced

½ pound fresh mozzarella, sliced

1½ cups lower-sodium marinara

½ cup fresh basil leaves, torn

1. Preheat the oven to 425°F.

2. Coat the eggplant slices in 1 tablespoon olive oil and sprinkle with the salt and black pepper. Place on a large baking sheet and roast for 10 to 12 minutes, until soft with crispy edges. Remove the eggplant and set the oven to a low broil.

3. In a bowl, stir together the remaining tablespoon of olive oil, bread crumbs, Parmesan cheese, and garlic.

4. Remove the cooled eggplant from the baking sheet and clean. Create layers on the same baking sheet by stacking a roasted eggplant slice with a slice of mozzarella, a tablespoon of marinara, and a tablespoon of the bread crumb mixture, repeating with 2 layers of each ingredient. Place under the broiler for 3 to 4 minutes, until the cheese is melted and bubbly.

SUBSTITUTION TIP: For a gluten-free version, use gluten-free panko bread crumbs.

COOKING TIP: To avoid a watery stack, sprinkle salt on the raw eggplant, let it sit for 10 minutes, then dry it with a paper towel before cooking.

VARIATION TIP: Try grilling the eggplant instead of roasting. Follow the same method and cook time while cooking on a grill pan or outdoor grill.

MAKE IT A MEAL: Serve with a side of grilled, roasted, or sautéed vegetables or fresh fruit.

PER SERVING: Total Calories: 377; Total Fat: 22g; Saturated Fat: 10g; Cholesterol: 44mg; Sodium: 509mg; Potassium: 397mg; Total Carbohydrate: 29g; Fiber: 6g; Sugars: 11g; Protein: 16g

Roasted Vegetable Enchiladas

VEGETARIAN • MEAL-IN-ONE

SERVES 8   PREP TIME: 25 MINUTES   COOK TIME: 45 MINUTES

The roasted vegetables in this dish add a depth of flavor from the caramelization process, and the homemade enchilada sauce provides the smokiness of chipotle chiles. If you're not in the mood to turn on the oven, serve the veggies and sauce on a burrito bowl with rice, Greek yogurt, cilantro, and avocado.

2 zucchinis, diced

1 red bell pepper, seeded and sliced

1 red onion, peeled and sliced

2 ears corn

2 tablespoons canola oil

1 (15-ounce) can no-salt-added black beans, rinsed and drained

1½ tablespoons chili powder

2 teaspoon ground cumin

⅛ teaspoon kosher or sea salt

½ teaspoon ground black pepper

8 (8-inch) whole-wheat tortillas

1 cup Enchilada Sauce (page 220) or store-bought enchilada sauce

½ cup shredded Mexican-style cheese

½ cup plain nonfat Greek yogurt

½ cup cilantro leaves, chopped

1. Preheat oven to 400°F.

2. Place the zucchini, red bell pepper, and red onion together on a baking sheet. Place the ears of corn separately on the same baking sheet. Drizzle all with the canola oil and toss to coat. Roast for 10 to 12 minutes, until the vegetables are tender. Remove from the oven and reduce the temperature to 375°F.

3. Cut the corn from the cob. Transfer the corn kernels, zucchini, red bell pepper, and onion to a bowl and stir in the black beans, chili powder, cumin, salt, and black pepper until combined.

4. Coat a 9-by-13-inch baking dish with cooking spray. Line up the tortillas in the greased baking dish. Evenly distribute the vegetable bean filling into each tortilla. Pour half of the enchilada sauce and sprinkle half of the shredded cheese on top of the filling. Roll each tortilla into enchilada shape and place them seam-side down. Pour the remaining enchilada sauce and sprinkle the remaining cheese over the enchiladas. Bake for 25 minutes, until the cheese is melted and bubbly.

5. Serve the enchiladas with Greek yogurt and chopped cilantro.

SUBSTITUTION TIP: For a meat version, try cooked chicken breast or cooked lean ground beef as a substitute for the black beans.

COOKING TIP: You can sauté the vegetables instead of roasting for a quicker version. Heat the oil in a large skillet and sauté the vegetables for 4 to 5 minutes, until slightly soft.

VARIATION TIP: Try summer squash, a rainbow of bell peppers, or jicama for the filling instead of the other vegetables.

PER SERVING: Total Calories: 335; Total Fat: 15g; Saturated Fat: 6g; Cholesterol: 19mg; Sodium: 557mg; Potassium: 289mg; Total Carbohydrate: 42g; Fiber: 7g; Sugars: 4g; Protein: 13g

Lentil Avocado Tacos

VEGAN · MEAL-IN-ONE

SERVES 6   PREP TIME: 10 MINUTES   COOK TIME: 35 MINUTES

For meatless meals, lentils are often a substitute because they're filled with protein and fiber, so they're filling. Plus, they're hearty, so they make a great base for taco meat, burgers, casseroles, and soups. Use the cooked, canned variety for an even quicker meal.

1 tablespoon canola oil

½ yellow onion, peeled and diced

2 to 3 garlic cloves, peeled
    and minced

1½ cups dried lentils

½ teaspoon kosher or sea salt

3 to 3½ cups unsalted vegetable or
    chicken stock

2½ tablespoons Taco Seasoning
    (page 216) or store-bought low-
    sodium taco seasoning

16 (6-inch) corn tortillas, toasted

2 ripe avocados, peeled and sliced

1. Heat the canola oil in a large skillet or Dutch oven over medium heat. Add the onion and sauté for 4 to 5 minutes, until soft. Stir in the garlic and cook for 30 seconds until fragrant. Then add the lentils, salt, and stock. Bring to a simmer for 25 to 35 minutes, adding additional stock if needed.

2. When there's only a small amount of liquid left in the pan and the lentils are al dente, stir in the taco seasoning and let simmer for 1 to 2 minutes. Taste and adjust the seasoning, if necessary.

3. Spoon the lentil mixture into tortillas and serve with the avocado slices.

4. Store leftover lentil mixture in airtight containers in the refrigerator for up to 5 days. Reheat in the microwave for 1 to 2 minutes, until heated through.

COOKING TIP: Canned (cooked) lentils can be substituted for dried. Simply add them to the sautéed onion, add only ½ cup of stock, and add the seasoning. Let the mixture simmer for a few minutes, until heated through.

VARIATION TIP: Make a burrito bowl with the lentil taco "meat." Pack the bowls with cooked rice or quinoa, lentil taco "meat," avocado, cilantro, and plain nonfat Greek yogurt.

PER SERVING: Total Calories: 400; Total Fat: 14g; Saturated Fat: 1g; Cholesterol: 0mg; Sodium: 336mg; Potassium: 631mg; Total Carbohydrate: 64g; Fiber: 15g; Sugars: 3g; Protein: 16g

Tomato & Olive Orecchiette with Basil Pesto

VEGAN • MEAL-IN-ONE

SERVES 6   PREP TIME: 15 MINUTES   COOK TIME: 25 MINUTES

Orecchiette is an ear-shaped pasta that is hearty and acts as a vehicle for whatever sauce it's paired with. Any Mediterranean-style ingredients work well in this dish. You can add artichoke hearts, roasted red peppers, and fresh mozzarella if you would like.

12 ounces orecchiette pasta

2 tablespoons olive oil

1 pint cherry tomatoes, quartered

½ cup Basil Pesto (page 212) or store-bought pesto

¼ cup kalamata olives, sliced

1 tablespoon dried oregano leaves

¼ teaspoon kosher or sea salt

½ teaspoon freshly cracked black pepper

¼ teaspoon crushed red pepper flakes

2 tablespoons freshly grated Parmesan cheese

1. Bring a large pot of water to a boil. Add the orecchiette and cook according to the package directions. Drain and transfer the pasta to a large nonstick skillet.

2. Place the skillet over medium-low heat and heat the olive oil. Stir in the cherry tomatoes, pesto, olives, oregano, salt, black pepper, and crushed red pepper flakes. Cook, stirring frequently, for 8 to 10 minutes, until heated throughout.

3. Serve the pasta with the freshly grated Parmesan cheese.

4. For leftovers, divide the pasta into microwaveable airtight containers and refrigerate for up to 5 days. Reheat in the microwave on high for 1½ to 2 minutes, until heated through.

SUBSTITUTION TIP: Instead of orecchiette, use bow tie, penne, or elbow macaroni, if desired.

VARIATION TIP: This pasta can be served cold as a salad, too. Chill it after cooking and add additional olive oil if it becomes a bit dry.

MAKE IT A MEAL: Add cooked tofu or chicken for a higher-protein meal.

PER SERVING: Total Calories: 332; Total Fat: 13g; Saturated Fat: 2g; Cholesterol: 1mg; Sodium: 389mg; Potassium: 125mg; Total Carbohydrate: 44g; Fiber: 2g; Sugars: 1g; Protein: 9g

Italian Stuffed Portobello Mushroom Burgers

SERVES 4   PREP TIME: 20 MINUTES   COOK TIME: 25 MINUTES

Mushrooms provide a hearty dose of umami when cooked, making them a favorite among vegetarians and meat eaters. That flavor is imparted in these roasted burgers that are stuffed with Italian-style ingredients and served on a bun with fresh arugula. The bean stuffing provides DASH-friendly protein and fiber.

1 tablespoon olive oil

4 large portobello mushrooms, washed and dried

½ yellow onion, peeled and diced

4 garlic cloves, peeled and minced

1 (15-ounce) can cannellini beans, drained and rinsed

½ cup fresh basil leaves, torn

½ cup panko bread crumbs

⅛ teaspoon kosher or sea salt

¼ teaspoon ground black pepper

1 cup lower-sodium marinara, divided

½ cup shredded mozzarella cheese

4 whole-wheat buns, toasted

1 cup fresh arugula

1. Heat the olive oil in a large skillet to medium-high heat. Sear the mushrooms for 4 to 5 minutes per side, until slightly soft. Place on a baking sheet.

2. Preheat the oven to a low broil.

3. Place the onion in the skillet and cook for 4 to 5 minutes, until slightly soft. Stir in the garlic and cook until fragrant, 30 to 60 seconds. Transfer the onions and garlic to a bowl. Add the cannellini beans and smash with the back of a fork to form a chunky paste. Stir in the basil, bread crumbs, salt, and black pepper and half of the marinara. Cook for 5 minutes.

4. Remove the bean mixture from the stove and divide among the mushroom caps. Spoon the remaining marinara over the stuffed mushrooms and top each with the mozzarella cheese. Broil for 3 to 4 minutes, until the cheese is melted and bubbly.

5. Transfer the burgers to the toasted whole-wheat buns and top with the arugula.

SUBSTITUTION TIP: For a vegan version, replace mozzarella with vegan mozzarella.

COOKING TIP: Wash the portobello mushrooms by dampening a paper towel and wiping them out. If you run them under water, they may become watery and soggy when cooked. Do not wash them until just before use.

VARIATION TIP: Skip the bun and eat these stuffed portobello burgers with a fork!

PER SERVING: Total Calories: 407; Total Fat: 9g; Saturated Fat: 2g; Cholesterol: 8mg; Sodium: 575mg; Potassium: 77mg; Total Carbohydrate: 63g; Fiber: 14g; Sugars: 12g; Protein: 25g

Gnocchi with Tomato Basil Sauce

VEGETARIAN · MEAL-IN-ONE

SERVES 6   PREP TIME: 15 MINUTES   COOK TIME: 25 MINUTES

Gnocchi are small potato dumplings traditionally used in Italian dishes. They cook in about 5 minutes and hold up well with thick, hearty sauces. Our version is served with a simple, light tomato basil sauce made with sweet San Marzano tomatoes.

2 tablespoons olive oil

½ yellow onion, peeled and diced

3 cloves garlic, peeled and minced

1 (32-ounce) can no-salt-added crushed San Marzano tomatoes

¼ cup fresh basil leaves

2 teaspoons Italian seasoning

½ teaspoon kosher or sea salt

1 teaspoon granulated sugar

½ teaspoon ground black pepper

⅛ teaspoon crushed red pepper flakes

1 tablespoon heavy cream (optional)

12 ounces gnocchi

¼ cup freshly grated Parmesan cheese

1. Heat the olive oil in a Dutch oven or stockpot over medium heat. Add the onion and sauté for 5 to 6 minutes, until soft. Stir in the garlic and stir until fragrant, 30 to 60 seconds. Then stir in the tomatoes, basil, Italian seasoning, salt, sugar, black pepper, and crushed red pepper flakes. Bring to a simmer for 15 minutes. Stir in the heavy cream, if desired.

For a smooth, puréed sauce, use an immersion blender or transfer sauce to a blender and purée until smooth. Taste and adjust the seasoning, if necessary.

2. While the sauce simmers, cook the gnocchi according the package instructions, remove with a slotted spoon, and transfer to 6 bowls. Pour the sauce over the gnocchi and top with the Parmesan cheese.

SUBSTITUTION TIP: For a vegan version, omit the Parmesan cheese or use nutritional yeast flakes as a topping.

COOKING TIP: When puréeing a hot mixture in a blender, remove the small cap on the lid and hold a kitchen towel down over it so some of the steam can escape. If the lid is fully closed, the top could explode once you turn the blender on.

MAKE IT A MEAL: Serve with a side of grilled, sautéed, or roasted vegetables.

PER SERVING: Total Calories: 287; Total Fat: 7g; Saturated Fat: 1g; Cholesterol: 40mg; Sodium: 527mg; Potassium: 32mg; Total Carbohydrate: 41g; Fiber: 9g; Sugars: 5g; Protein: 10g

Creamy Pumpkin Pasta

SERVES 6   PREP TIME: 15 MINUTES   COOK TIME: 30 MINUTES

Adding starchy pasta water to the sauce in this recipe makes it thick, creamy, and luxurious. With notes of nutmeg, sage, and garlic, this pumpkin sauce will become your new favorite to toss with pasta, especially when the temperature begins to drop outside.

1 pound whole-grain linguine

1 tablespoon olive oil

3 garlic cloves, peeled and minced

2 tablespoons chopped fresh sage

1½ cups pumpkin purée

1 cup unsalted vegetable stock

½ cup low-fat evaporated milk

¾ teaspoon kosher or sea salt

½ teaspoon ground black pepper

½ teaspoon ground nutmeg

¼ teaspoon ground cayenne pepper

½ cup freshly grated Parmesan cheese, divided

1. Bring a large pot of water to a boil. Cook the whole-grain linguine according to the package directions. Reserve ½ cup of pasta water and drain the rest. Set the pasta aside.

2. In a large skillet, heat the olive oil over medium heat. Add the garlic and sage and sauté for 1 to 2 minutes, until soft and fragrant. Whisk in the pumpkin purée, stock, milk, and reserved pasta water and simmer for 4 to 5 minutes, until thickened. Whisk in the salt, black pepper, nutmeg, and cayenne pepper and half of the Parmesan cheese. Stir in the cooked whole-grain linguine.

3. Evenly divide the pasta among 6 bowls and top with the remaining Parmesan cheese.

4. For leftovers, transfer the pasta into microwaveable airtight containers and refrigerate for up to 5 days. Reheat in the microwave on high for 1 to 3 minutes, until heated through.

COOKING TIP: Evaporated milk is a good substitute for heavy cream in soups and pasta sauces. It is still thick and creamy, but it is much lower in fat.

VARIATION TIP: Try using cooked butternut squash instead of pumpkin.

MAKE IT A MEAL: For a higher-protein meat version, add cooked ground turkey sausage.

PER SERVING: Total Calories: 381; Total Fat: 8g; Saturated Fat: 2g; Cholesterol: 6mg; Sodium: 175mg; Potassium: 300mg; Total Carbohydrate: 63g; Fiber: 10g; Sugars: 7g; Protein: 15g

Mexican-Style Potato Casserole

VEGETARIAN

SERVES 8   PREP TIME: 25 MINUTES   COOK TIME: 1 HOUR

This casserole is a spicy take on potatoes au gratin. It's comfort food but a much healthier version, with lower-fat ingredients, loads of potatoes, and plenty of flavor from the spices and green chiles. While the casserole bakes, whip up some grilled or sautéed vegetables as a side dish or a bowl of fresh fruit.

Cooking spray

2 tablespoons canola oil

½ yellow onion, peeled and diced

4 garlic cloves, peeled and minced

2 tablespoons all-purpose flour

1¼ cups milk

1 tablespoon chili powder

½ tablespoon ground cumin

1 teaspoon kosher salt or sea salt

½ teaspoon ground black pepper

¼ teaspoon ground cayenne pepper

1½ cups shredded Mexican-style cheese, divided

1 (4-ounce) can green chiles, drained

1½ pounds baby Yukon Gold or red potatoes, thinly sliced

1 red bell pepper, thinly sliced

1. Preheat the oven to 400°F. Coat a 9-by-13-inch baking dish with cooking spray.

2. In a large saucepan, heat the canola oil over medium heat. Add the onion and sauté for 4 to 5 minutes, until soft. Stir in the garlic and cook until fragrant, 30 to 60 seconds. Whisk in the flour to create a roux, then slowly pour in the milk while whisking. Bring to a slow simmer for about 5 minutes, until thickened. Whisk in the chili powder, cumin, salt, black pepper, and cayenne pepper. Remove from the heat and whisk in half of the shredded cheese and the green chiles. Taste and adjust the seasoning, if necessary.

3. Line up one-third of the sliced potatoes and sliced bell pepper in the baking dish and top with quarter of the remaining shredded cheese. Repeat with 2 more layers. Pour the cheese sauce over the top and sprinkle with the remaining shredded cheese.

4. Cover the baking dish with aluminum foil and bake for 45 to 50 minutes, until the potatoes are tender. Remove the foil and bake for an additional 5 to 10 minutes, until the topping is slightly browned. Let cool for 20 minutes before slicing into 8 pieces.

5. Transfer slices of the casserole to microwaveable airtight containers and refrigerate for up to 5 days. Reheat in the microwave on high for 2 to 3 minutes, until heated through.

SUBSTITUTION TIP: For a gluten-free version, replace all-purpose flour with gluten-free all-purpose flour.

COOKING TIP: You can use a standard chef's knife to thinly slice potatoes, or, if you prefer, you can use a mandoline with the hand guard to evenly and quickly slice potatoes.

VARIATION TIP: Replace regular potatoes with sweet potatoes.

PER SERVING: Total Calories: 195; Total Fat: 10g; Saturated Fat: 4g; Cholesterol: 19mg; Sodium: 487mg; Potassium: 489mg; Total Carbohydrate: 19g; Fiber: 2g; Sugars: 4g; Protein: 8g

Black Bean Stew with Cornbread

VEGETARIAN · MEAL-IN-ONE

SERVES 6   PREP TIME: 20 MINUTES   COOK TIME: 55 MINUTES

This black bean stew is loaded with onion, garlic, and cumin. The diced tomatoes add a burst of roasted flavor to the dish. The buttermilk honey cornbread topping is light and fluffy and turns a stew into a home-run casserole. It's perfect to make ahead and reheat for quick weeknight meals.

FOR THE BLACK BEAN STEW:

2 tablespoons canola oil

1 yellow onion, peeled and diced

4 garlic cloves, peeled and minced

1 tablespoon chili powder

1 tablespoon ground cumin

¼ teaspoon kosher or sea salt

½ teaspoon ground black pepper

2 (15-ounce) cans no-salt-added black
   beans, rinsed and drained

1 (10-ounce) can fire-roasted diced
   tomatoes

½ cup fresh cilantro leaves, chopped

FOR THE CORNBREAD TOPPING:

1¼ cups cornmeal

½ cup all-purpose flour

½ teaspoon baking powder

¼ teaspoon baking soda

⅛ teaspoon kosher or sea salt

1 cup low-fat buttermilk

2 tablespoons honey

1 large egg

TO MAKE THE BLACK BEAN STEW:

In a large Dutch oven or stockpot, heat the canola oil over medium heat. Add the onion and sauté for 4 to 6 minutes, until the onion is soft. Stir in the garlic, chili powder, cumin, salt, and black pepper. Cook for 1 to 2 minutes, until fragrant. Add the black beans and diced tomatoes. Bring to a simmer and cook for 15 minutes. Remove from the heat and stir in the fresh cilantro. Taste and adjust the seasoning, if necessary.

TO MAKE THE CORNBREAD TOPPING:

1. Preheat the oven to 375°F.

2. While the stew simmers, prepare the cornbread topping. In a bowl, whisk together the cornmeal, flour, baking powder, baking soda, and salt until combined. In a measuring cup, whisk together the buttermilk, honey, and egg until combined. Fold the mixture into the dry ingredients until just combined.

3. In oven-safe bowls or dishes, spoon out the black bean soup. Next, distribute dollops of the cornbread batter on top and then spread it out evenly with a spatula. Bake for 30 minutes, until the cornbread is just set.

SUBSTITUTION TIP: To make the cornbread topping vegan, substitute 1 cup almond or soy milk plus 1 teaspoon white vinegar for the buttermilk, and leave out the honey.

COOKING TIP: Add spices and herbs to the pot before adding any beans or liquid to help release their oils and impart more flavor to the final stew.

VARIATION TIP: Try using pinto beans instead of black beans.

PER SERVING: Total Calories: 359; Total Fat: 7g; Saturated Fat: 1g; Cholesterol: 37mg; Sodium: 409mg; Potassium: 408mg; Total Carbohydrate: 61g; Fiber: 10g; Sugars: 11g; Protein: 14g

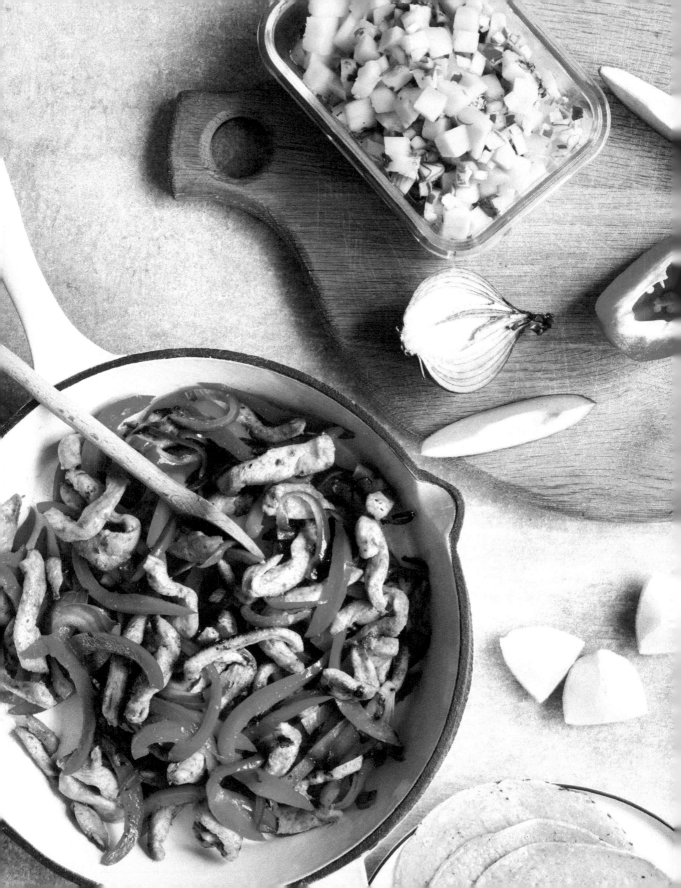

Seafood and Poultry Mains

Grilled Salmon with Chimichurri

SERVES 4 PREP TIME: 15 MINUTES   COOK TIME: 10 MINUTES

Salmon is a great source of omega-3 fatty acids, which are important for heart and brain health. Due to its high fat content, it goes well with a light herb sauce like chimichurri. This meal comes together in less than 30 minutes and is bursting with fresh flavors.

FOR THE CHIMICHURRI:

½ cup fresh flat-leaf Italian parsley leaves

¼ cup fresh cilantro leaves

½ jalapeño, seeded

4 cloves garlic, peeled

¼ cup red wine vinegar

2 tablespoons olive oil

1 teaspoon honey

1 teaspoon dried oregano leaves

½ teaspoon kosher or sea salt

¼ teaspoon ground black pepper

FOR THE GRILLED SALMON:

4 (4-ounce) salmon fillets, skin on

1 tablespoon olive oil

2 teaspoons chili powder

⅛ teaspoon kosher or sea salt

⅛ teaspoon ground black pepper

TO MAKE THE CHIMICHURRI:

Place all the chimichurri ingredients in a food processor and pulse until a pesto-like consistency is reached. Taste and adjust the seasoning, if necessary.

Spoon into an airtight container and place in your refrigerator.

TO MAKE THE GRILLED SALMON:

1. Preheat the grill to medium. Rub the salmon fillets with the olive oil and season with the chili powder, salt, and black pepper. Place the fillets on the grill, skin-side down, and cook about 10 minutes, until the fish flakes easily with a fork.

2. Serve the chimichurri over the grilled salmon fillets.

SUBSTITUTION TIP: Use any whitefish instead of salmon, if desired.

VARIATION TIP: Try fresh oregano instead of fresh cilantro in the chimichurri for a unique flavor.

MAKE IT A MEAL: Serve with grilled vegetables and Fluffy Brown Rice (page 223).

PER SERVING: Total Calories: 341; Total Fat: 25g; Saturated Fat: 5g; Cholesterol: 70mg; Sodium: 532mg; Potassium: 127mg; Total Carbohydrate: 4g; Fiber: 1g; Sugars: 2g; Protein: 26g

Almond-Crusted Tuna Cakes

SERVES 4   PREP TIME: 15 MINUTES   COOK TIME: 15 MINUTES

Canned tuna is packed with protein and is already cooked, so it's a simple and quick ingredient to add to pasta, casseroles, or salads for a satisfying meal. Some canned tuna is high in sodium, so it's best to compare nutrition labels and choose a lower-sodium version.

½ cup almonds

9 ounces canned albacore tuna

2 large eggs

½ cup panko bread crumbs

¼ cup fresh parsley leaves, chopped

Zest and juice of ½ lemon

1 tablespoon Dijon mustard

1 teaspoon Italian seasoning

¼ teaspoon kosher or sea salt

¼ teaspoon ground black pepper

2 tablespoons olive oil

1. Place almonds in a food processor and pulse until crumbly. Transfer to a shallow dish.

2. Clean the food processor. Put the tuna, eggs, bread crumbs, parsley, lemon zest and juice, Dijon mustard, Italian seasoning, salt, and black pepper in the food processor and pulse until a paste forms, scraping down the sides of the processor bowl as needed. Form the mixture into 4 cakes. Press the patties into the crushed almonds on all sides.

3. Heat the olive oil in a skillet over medium heat. Place the cakes in the hot oil and fry for 3 minutes on each side, until browned and crispy.

4. For leftovers, place in microwaveable airtight containers for 3 to 4 days. Reheat in the microwave on high for 1 to 2 minutes, until heated through.

SUBSTITUTION TIP: Substitute canned crab for canned tuna, if desired.

COOKING TIP: You can also cook the cakes in the oven. Place them on a baking sheet and roast at 400°F for 10 minutes.

VARIATION TIP: Replace almonds with walnuts, sunflower seeds, or pepitas.

MAKE IT A MEAL: Serve with a salad or roasted, sautéed, or grilled vegetables to make it a meal.

PER SERVING: Total Calories: 293; Total Fat: 19g; Saturated Fat: 3g; Cholesterol: 124mg; Sodium: 435mg; Potassium: 324mg; Total Carbohydrate: 11g; Fiber: 3g; Sugars: 1g; Protein: 20g

Spinach & Feta Salmon Burgers

MEAL-IN-ONE · UNDER 30 MINUTES

SERVES 4   PREP TIME: 10 MINUTES   COOK TIME: 20 MINUTES

Salmon burgers are the perfect way to enjoy a favorite while adding in a boost of heart-healthy fats. This version has Greek-inspired ingredients like feta, spinach, dill, cucumbers, tomato, and Greek yogurt. The entire meal takes about a half hour to make, and can easily be served throughout the week.

1 pound salmon fillets, skin removed

1 cup fresh spinach, chopped

½ cup panko bread crumbs

¼ cup crumbled feta cheese

1 large egg

1 tablespoon Dijon mustard

½ teaspoon dried dill

¼ teaspoon kosher or sea salt

¼ teaspoon ground black pepper

½ cup plain nonfat Greek yogurt

½ English cucumber, sliced

1 beefsteak tomato, sliced

1. Preheat the oven to 400°F. Line a baking sheet with parchment paper.

2. Place the salmon in the bowl of a food processor and pulse until ground. Transfer to a bowl and stir in the spinach, bread crumbs, feta cheese, egg, Dijon mustard, dill, salt, and black pepper until well combined. Use your hands to form 4 burger-size patties. Place them on the parchment paper and bake for 20 minutes, until the internal temperature reaches 145°F.

3. Serve the burgers with dollops of the Greek yogurt and slices of the cucumber and tomato.

4. For leftovers, place the burgers in microwaveable airtight containers for up to 3 to 4 days. Reheat in the microwave on high for 2 to 3 minutes, until heated through. Assemble the burgers before consuming.

SUBSTITUTION TIP: For a fish-free version, use ground turkey or chicken instead of the salmon.

COOKING TIP: The salmon patties can also be cooked on the stove. Heat a tablespoon of oil in a grill pan or skillet over medium heat. Add the patties and sauté for 4 to 5 minutes per side.

VARIATION TIP: Replace the salmon with whitefish, such as cod, halibut, or haddock, if desired.

PER SERVING: Total Calories: 238; Total Fat: 8g; Saturated Fat: 2g; Cholesterol: 109mg; Sodium: 453mg; Potassium: 106mg; Total Carbohydrate: 10g; Fiber: 1g; Sugars: 3g; Protein: 30g

Crispy Balsamic Chicken Thighs

SERVES 4   PREP TIME: 10 MINUTES   COOK TIME: 20 MINUTES

A delightfully tangy and sweet sauce makes the perfect finish for seared chicken thighs. Serve with vegetables, soup, or a grain side dish for a family favorite weeknight meal that is ready in less than 30 minutes.

¼ cup balsamic vinegar

2 tablespoons honey

1 tablespoon low-sodium soy sauce

3 cloves garlic, peeled and minced

1 tablespoon canola oil

**1 pound boneless skinless
   chicken thighs**

¼ teaspoon kosher or sea salt

¼ teaspoon ground black pepper

1. Preheat the oven to 375°F.

2. In a small bowl, whisk together the balsamic vinegar, honey, soy sauce, and garlic until combined.

3. Heat the canola oil in an oven-safe skillet to medium-high. Season the chicken thighs with the salt and black pepper. Once the pan is hot, place the chicken thighs into the pan and sear until crispy, about 5 minutes. Turn the chicken over and cook another 2 to 3 minutes. Add the sauce to the pan and bring to a simmer. Transfer to the oven and roast for 10 minutes, until the internal temperature reaches 165°F.

4. Serve immediately or place in microwaveable airtight containers and refrigerate for up to 5 days. To reheat, microwave on high for 1 to 2 minutes, until heated through.

SUBSTITUTION TIP: For a gluten-free version, use low-sodium tamari instead of soy sauce.

COOKING TIP: When searing meat, leave it untouched in a medium-high skillet until the bottom is lightly browned and crispy. If you turn or move the meat too frequently, the brown crust will not form.

VARIATION TIP: Instead of the chicken thighs, try lean 4-ounce steaks.

PER SERVING: Total Calories: 227; Total Fat: 10g; Saturated Fat: 2g; Cholesterol: 65mg; Sodium: 385mg; Potassium: 14mg; Total Carbohydrate: 12g; Fiber: 0g; Sugars: 9g; Protein: 21g

Shrimp Noodle Bowls with Ginger Broth

SERVES 6 PREP TIME: 15 MINUTES COOK TIME: 35 MINUTES

Noodle bowls are all the rage, and for good reason. The broth is loaded with ginger, garlic, and chili flavors. The bowls are filled with succulent shrimp, crisp vegetables, and perfectly al dente brown rice noodles. This recipe comes together in no time and is a wonderfully delicious Asian-influenced meal.

FOR THE BROTH:

1 pound shrimp, deveined and divided

2 cups unsalted fish stock

2-inch piece ginger, peeled and sliced

2 teaspoons chili garlic sauce

½ teaspoon kosher or sea salt

½ teaspoon ground black pepper

FOR THE NOODLE BOWLS:

8 ounces brown rice noodles

1 tablespoon canola oil

½ yellow onion, peeled and thinly sliced

1 red bell pepper, seeded and thinly sliced

1 cup sugar snap peas, thinly sliced

4 garlic cloves, peeled and minced

¼ teaspoon kosher or sea salt

½ cup fresh cilantro leaves (optional)

TO MAKE THE BROTH:

Peel the shrimp and place the shells in a large pot. Set the peeled shrimp aside. Add the fish stock, ginger, chili garlic sauce, salt, and black pepper to the pot and bring to a simmer for 15 minutes.

TO MAKE THE NOODLE BOWLS:

1. While the broth is simmering, bring a large pot of water to a boil. Cook the noodles according to the package directions.

2. In that same pot, heat the canola oil to medium. Add the yellow onion, red bell pepper, and snap peas and sauté for 4 to 5 minutes, until the vegetables are slightly soft. Add the shrimp and cook for 2 to 3 minutes, then stir in the garlic and salt.

3. Divide the noodles and shrimp mixture into 6 bowls and pour the broth into each bowl. Top with the cilantro, if desired.

SUBSTITUTION TIP: If you can't find brown rice noodles, you can use whole-grain spaghetti.

COOKING TIP: For a richer, more flavorful broth, simmer for up to an hour.

VARIATION TIP: Use chicken or salmon instead of the shrimp, if desired.

PER SERVING: Total Calories: 272; Total Fat: 5g; Saturated Fat: 1g; Cholesterol: 115mg; Sodium: 430mg; Potassium: 200mg; Total Carbohydrate: 36g; Fiber: 4g; Sugars: 3g; Protein: 20g

Shrimp Pasta Primavera

SERVES 6   PREP TIME: 20 MINUTES   COOK TIME: 40 MINUTES

A meal like pasta primavera seems like it belongs in a fancy bistro, but it's easy to make right in your own kitchen! With juicy shrimp, colorful veggies, and tender pasta, you'll surely be satisfied. And it's the perfect dish to pack up in containers and reheat the next day.

12 ounces whole-grain spaghetti

1½ tablespoons unsalted butter

1 small head broccoli, chopped

1 red bell pepper, seeded and chopped

1 pound raw shrimp, deveined and shelled

1 cup frozen green peas

1 cup baby spinach leaves

5 garlic cloves, peeled and minced

¾ teaspoon kosher or sea salt

½ teaspoon ground black pepper

¼ teaspoon crushed red pepper flakes

Zest and juice of 1 lemon

½ cup unsalted vegetable, chicken, or fish stock

½ cup freshly grated Parmesan cheese

¼ cup fresh flat-leaf Italian parsley, chopped

1. Bring a large pot of water to a boil. Cook the spaghetti according to the package directions. Reserve ¼ cup of pasta water and drain the rest.

2. In a Dutch oven or large pot, heat the butter over medium heat. Add the broccoli and red bell pepper and sauté for 2 to 3 minutes, until slightly soft. Add the shrimp, green peas, and spinach and sauté for 2 to 3 minutes, until the shrimp is opaque. Stir in the garlic, salt, black pepper, and crushed red pepper flakes. Cook until fragrant.

3. Add the reserved pasta water, lemon zest and juice, and stock and bring to a simmer for 6 to 8 minutes, until thickened, stirring frequently.

4. Remove from the heat and stir in the Parmesan cheese and parsley. Taste and adjust the seasoning, if necessary.

5. For leftovers, divide the pasta into microwaveable airtight containers for up to 3 to 4 days. Reheat in the microwave for 2 to 3 minutes, until heated through.

SUBSTITUTION TIP: To make this recipe vegetarian, substitute 2 cups sliced mushrooms for the shrimp.

COOKING TIP: Acidic ingredients such as lemon juice or vinegar can provide a slightly salty flavor to a dish. Use them to cut back on the salt without sacrificing flavor.

VARIATION TIP: Instead of using broccoli, bell peppers, and peas, try a Mediterranean version with roasted red peppers, sun-dried tomatoes, and kalamata olives.

PER SERVING: Total Calories: 369; Total Fat: 7g; Saturated Fat: 2g; Cholesterol: 125mg; Sodium: 546mg; Potassium: 469mg; Total Carbohydrate: 43g; Fiber: 9g; Sugars: 5g; Protein: 30g

Indian-Spiced Chicken Kebabs

SERVES 4   PREP TIME: 20 MINUTES   COOK TIME: 15 MINUTES PLUS AT LEAST 30 MINUTES REFRIGERATION

With just a little marinating time, these Middle Eastern–inspired kebabs are an easy and quick way to get dinner on the table. They sing with lemon, garlic, ginger, and spices, and are grilled to perfection with eggplant and tomatoes. Start marinating the night before and serve with a batch of rice or quinoa for a complete meal.

½ cup plain nonfat Greek yogurt

Zest and juice of 1 lemon

4 garlic cloves, peeled and minced

1-inch piece fresh ginger, peeled and minced

2 tablespoons Garam Masala (page 215) or store-bought garam masala

¼ teaspoon kosher or sea salt, divided

¼ teaspoon ground cayenne pepper

1 pound boneless skinless chicken breasts, cubed

½ eggplant, cubed

1 pint cherry tomatoes, halved

1 tablespoon olive oil

1. In a large zip-top plastic bag, combine the greek yogurt, lemon zest and juice, garlic, ginger, and garam masala with half of the salt and the cayenne pepper. Shake the bag with your hands to mix. Add the chicken cubes to the bag, seal, and place in the refrigerator for at least 30 minutes or overnight.

2. Place the cubed eggplant and tomatoes in a small bowl, toss with the olive oil, and sprinkle with the remaining salt.

3. Preheat the grill or grill pan over medium-high heat. Thread the marinated chicken, cubed eggplant, and tomatoes on skewers. Discard the extra marinade. Grill the kebabs for 15 to 18 minutes, turning regularly, until the chicken reaches 165°F and the vegetables are soft and crispy.

SUBSTITUTION TIP: To make this vegetarian, substitute cauliflower for the chicken. Be sure to partially cook the cauliflower before threading on the skewers. Do this by steaming for 5 to 6 minutes, until slightly softened.

MAKE IT A MEAL: Serve with cooked brown rice, quinoa, or whole-wheat couscous for a complete meal.

PER SERVING: Total Calories: 215; Total Fat: 7g; Saturated Fat: 2g; Cholesterol: 71mg; Sodium: 522mg; Potassium: 407mg; Total Carbohydrate: 13g; Fiber: 3g; Sugars: 4g; Protein: 26g

Spaghetti & Chicken Meatballs

SERVES 8   PREP TIME: 20 MINUTES   COOK TIME: 30 MINUTES

These meatballs are leaner than traditional beef and pork meatballs but are packed with flavor and moisture from Dijon mustard. The whole-grain pasta provides fiber while the premade marinara makes meal preparation a cinch. While the meatballs cook, boil the pasta and warm the marinara to save time in the kitchen.

2 pounds ground chicken

2 large eggs

½ cup panko bread crumbs

1 tablespoon freshly grated Parmesan cheese

1 tablespoon Dijon mustard

½ tablespoon Italian seasoning

½ teaspoon kosher or sea salt

½ teaspoon ground black pepper

⅛ teaspoon crushed red pepper flakes

12 ounces whole-grain spaghetti

1 (24-ounce) jar lower-sodium marinara sauce

1. Preheat the oven to 375°F. Fit a baking sheet with a wire rack and coat with cooking spray.

2. In a mixing bowl, mix the ground chicken, eggs, bread crumbs, Parmesan cheese, Dijon mustard, Italian seasoning, salt, black pepper, and red pepper flakes until thoroughly combined. Form into 2-inch balls and line up on the wire rack. Bake for 18 to 22 minutes, until the internal temperature reaches 165°F.

3. While the meatballs cook, bring a large pot of water to a boil. Cook the spaghetti according to the package directions.

4. Bring the marinara sauce to a simmer in a pot or a saucepan, stirring frequently. Serve the meatballs over the spaghetti and spoon the marinara sauce on top.

SUBSTITUTION TIP: For a gluten-free version, substitute gluten-free pasta and panko bread crumbs, and read the ingredient labels for the marinara sauce and Dijon mustard to be sure they're gluten free.

VARIATION TIP: Use lean ground beef or turkey instead of chicken.

MAKE IT A MEAL: Serve with roasted, sautéed, or grilled vegetables.

PER SERVING: Total Calories: 426; Total Fat: 15g; Saturated Fat: 3g; Cholesterol: 148mg; Sodium: 394mg; Potassium: 168mg; Total Carbohydrate: 40g; Fiber: 5g; Sugars: 5g; Protein: 29g

Chili Lime Chicken Fajitas with Mango Salsa

SERVES 4   PREP TIME: 20 MINUTES   COOK TIME: 20 MINUTES PLUS 30 MINUTES REFRIGERATION

Fajitas are a family favorite, and this version is quick and simple. The marinade is something you can make in just a few minutes. The mango salsa adds freshness, color, and loads of flavor while providing a boost of nutrition. Serving fajitas on corn tortillas is typically a healthier choice because they're whole grain and contain minimal ingredients.

FOR THE MANGO SALSA:

1 mango, peeled, pitted, and diced

½ jalapeño, seeded and finely minced

¼ red onion, peeled and finely diced

½ cup fresh cilantro leaves, chopped

Zest and juice of 2 limes

¼ teaspoon kosher or sea salt

¼ teaspoon ground black pepper

FOR THE CHICKEN FAJITAS:

1 pound boneless skinless chicken breasts, sliced into ½-inch strips

½ cup Chili Lime Marinade (page 213)

2 red bell peppers, seeded and sliced

1 red onion, peeled and sliced

8 (6-inch) corn tortillas, toasted

1 avocado, peeled and sliced

TO MAKE THE MANGO SALSA:

Combine the salsa ingredients in a bowl fitted with a lid and refrigerate until use.

TO MAKE THE CHICKEN FAJITAS:

1. Place the sliced chicken breast and marinade in a bowl fitted with a lid or in a large zip-top plastic bag, and shake to coat. Refrigerate for at least 30 minutes.

2. Heat a skillet over medium heat. Add the chicken and sauté for 3 to 4 minutes until opaque, then add the red bell pepper and onion and sauté for 3 to 4 more minutes, until the chicken is fully cooked and the bell peppers and onion are soft.

3. Scoop the chicken, bell peppers, and onion mixture onto the corn tortillas and top with the avocado and mango salsa.

4. For leftovers, store the chicken, bell pepper, and onion mixture in microwaveable airtight containers in the refrigerator for up to 5 days. Reheat the chicken in the microwave for 1 to 2 minutes, until heated through. Store the salsa in airtight containers in the refrigerator for up to 2 to 3 days.

SUBSTITUTION TIP: To make this vegetarian, try cubed sweet potato or black beans instead of the chicken.

COOKING TIP: Corn tortillas are best when toasted in a dry, hot pan on the stove until lightly browned on both sides.

VARIATION TIP: Instead of the mango, try pineapple, kiwi, or cantaloupe in the salsa.

PER SERVING: Total Calories: 414; Total Fat: 11g; Saturated Fat: 1g; Cholesterol: 70mg; Sodium: 458mg; Potassium: 487mg; Total Carbohydrate: 54g; Fiber: 6g; Sugars: 14g; Protein: 27g

Chicken Tortilla Casserole

SERVES 8   PREP TIME: 20 MINUTES   COOK TIME: 35 MINUTES

This casserole layers tortillas, seasoned ground chicken, and vegetables. The easy homemade enchilada sauce and cheese topped with cilantro, avocado, and creamy Greek yogurt really bring this dish to another level. And the best part: You can assemble it in just minutes, is easily customizable, and is something the whole family will love. It keeps well when cut into wedges and stored in airtight containers.

1 tablespoon canola oil

1 yellow onion, peeled and diced

1 red bell pepper, seeded and diced

½ jalapeño pepper, seeded and diced

2 pounds ground chicken

4 cloves garlic, peeled and minced

2 tablespoons Taco Seasoning (page 216)

8 (8-inch) whole-wheat flour tortillas

1 cup Enchilada Sauce (page 220) or store-bought enchilada sauce

¾ cup shredded Mexican-style cheese

1 avocado, peeled and diced

¼ cup nonfat plain Greek yogurt

¼ cup fresh cilantro leaves, chopped

1. Preheat the oven to 375°F. Coat a 9-by-9-inch baking dish with cooking spray.

2. Heat the canola oil in a skillet over medium heat. Add the onion, red bell pepper, and jalapeño pepper and sauté for 4 to 5 minutes, until soft. Add the ground chicken and sauté for another 5 to 7 minutes, stirring frequently while breaking up the meat, until chicken is cooked. Stir in the garlic and taco seasoning. Remove from the heat.

3. Line up 3 tortillas in the baking dish to cover the bottom, overlapping as needed. Layer with ⅓ of the meat, ⅓ of the sauce, and ⅓ of the cheese. Create another two layers, ending with shredded cheese. Bake for 20 minutes, until the cheese is melted and bubbly.

4. Slice into 8 wedges and top with the avocado, Greek yogurt, and cilantro.

5. Store leftovers in microwaveable airtight containers for up to 5 days. Reheat in the microwave on high for 2 to 3 minutes, until heated through.

SUBSTITUTION TIP: For a gluten-free version, try corn tortillas instead of whole wheat.

COOKING TIP: Keep a large batch of minced garlic on hand by adding several heads of peeled cloves in a small food processor and pulse until minced. Place in an airtight container or plastic bag and freeze.

VARIATION TIP: Use ground turkey or lean ground beef or pork instead of chicken, if desired.

PER SERVING: Total Calories: 376; Total Fat: 21g; Saturated Fat: 1g; Cholesterol: 109mg; Sodium: 535mg; Potassium: 179mg; Total Carbohydrate: 32g; Fiber: 5g; Sugars: 3g; Protein: 30g

Mexican-Style Turkey Stuffed Peppers

MEAL-IN-ONE

SERVES 6   PREP TIME: 15 MINUTES   COOK TIME: 1 HOUR 10 MINUTES

These bell peppers are stuffed with a seasoned turkey and black bean mixture and baked with gooey cheese on top. They're an easy way to get in several servings of vegetables and can be prepped and baked ahead of time.

6 red bell peppers, tops cut off

½ cup water

1 tablespoon canola oil

½ yellow onion, peeled and diced

1½ pounds ground turkey

4 garlic cloves, peeled and minced

2 tablespoons Taco Seasoning (page 216) or store-bought low-sodium taco seasoning

2 tablespoons no-salt-added tomato paste

½ teaspoon kosher or sea salt

1 (15-ounce) can fire-roasted petite diced tomatoes, drained

1 (15-ounce) can black beans, drained and rinsed

1 (4-ounce) can diced green chiles

½ cup fresh cilantro leaves, chopped

1 cup shredded Monterey Jack cheese

1. Preheat the oven to 375°F. Coat a baking dish with cooking spray. Place the peppers in the baking dish, pour ½ cup of water into the bottom of the dish, and cover with aluminum foil. Bake for 15 minutes and remove from the oven.

2. Heat the canola oil in a skillet over medium heat. Add the onion and ground turkey. Sauté for 7 to 10 minutes, until the turkey is browned. Stir in the garlic, taco seasoning, tomato paste, and salt. Add the diced tomatoes, black beans, and green chiles and bring to a simmer. Remove from the heat and stir in the cilantro. Taste and adjust the seasoning, if necessary.

3. Place the bell peppers in the baking dish. Fill each with the turkey black bean mixture. Bake uncovered for 35 to 40 minutes, until the peppers are tender. Top with the Monterey Jack cheese and bake for an additional 5 to 10 minutes, until the cheese is bubbly.

4. For leftovers, place in microwaveable airtight containers and reheat in the microwave on high for 2 to 3 minutes, until heated through.

SUBSTITUTION TIP: For a vegetarian version, replace the ground turkey with 2 cups cooked brown rice.

COOKING TIP: If the peppers do not stand up straight, slice a small amount off the bottom of each pepper so it is flat.

VARIATION TIP: Replace the taco seasoning with Italian seasoning, the black beans with cannellini, and the cilantro with parsley and omit the green chiles for Italian-inspired stuffed peppers.

PER SERVING: Total Calories: 374; Total Fat: 15g; Saturated Fat: 6g; Cholesterol: 95mg; Sodium: 528mg; Potassium: 418mg; Total Carbohydrate: 27g; Fiber: 7g; Sugars: 4g; Protein: 30g

Turkey Taco Weeknight Skillet

MEAL-IN-ONE • UNDER 30 MINUTES

SERVES 6   PREP TIME: 10 MINUTES   COOK TIME: 20 MINUTES

With just a few simple ingredients and a few minutes of prep, you can whip up this weeknight skillet in less than 30 minutes. The sweet potatoes and black beans provide fiber, and the turkey provides protein for a filling and satisfying dish. Use your favorite taco toppings to make it into a desirable and easy weeknight meal.

1 tablespoon canola oil

2 sweet potatoes, peeled and diced

1 pound ground turkey (93% lean)

1½ tablespoons Taco Seasoning (page 216)

¾ teaspoon kosher or sea salt

1 (15-ounce) can no-salt-added black beans

1 cup Simple Tomato Salsa (page 211) or store-bought fresh salsa

15 corn tortilla chips, crushed

1 avocado, peeled and diced

1 cup shredded lettuce

1. Heat the canola oil in a large skillet over medium heat. Add the diced sweet potato and cook, stirring frequently, for about 10 minutes, until slightly tender. Add the ground turkey and cook for 7 to 8 minutes, until the turkey is browned. Stir in the taco seasoning and salt.

2. Add the black beans and salsa to the skillet and bring to a simmer.

3. Remove from the stove and transfer to a bowl. Ladle into bowls and top with the crushed tortilla chips, diced avocados, and shredded lettuce.

4. For leftovers, divide into microwaveable airtight containers and refrigerate for up to 5 days. Reheat in the microwave on high for 2 to 3 minutes, until heated through.

SUBSTITUTION TIP: Swap in diced Yukon Gold or red potatoes instead of sweet potatoes.

COOKING TIP: For a quicker version, roast a large batch of diced sweet potatoes on the weekend and add them to the cooked ground turkey.

VARIATION TIP: Try lean ground beef or pork instead of turkey.

PER SERVING: Total Calories: 331; Total Fat: 14g; Saturated Fat: 3g; Cholesterol: 53mg; Sodium: 492mg; Potassium: 235mg; Total Carbohydrate: 31g; Fiber: 7g; Sugars: 6g; Protein: 20g

Italian-Style Turkey Meat Loaf

SERVES 8 **PREP TIME: 15 MINUTES** **COOK TIME: 50 MINUTES**

Good old meat loaf gets a flavor upgrade in this recipe by incorporating Italian seasoning, mozzarella cheese, and marinara sauce. Although turkey is a lean meat, this meat loaf is tender and juicy because it contains ingredients like Dijon mustard that provide moisture and flavor.

1½ pounds ground turkey

½ yellow onion, peeled and finely minced

5 garlic cloves, peeled and minced

2 large eggs

1 cup panko bread crumbs

½ cup fresh flat-leaf Italian parsley, chopped

1 tablespoon Dijon mustard

1 tablespoon Italian seasoning

¾ teaspoon kosher or sea salt

½ teaspoon ground black pepper

½ cup shredded mozzarella cheese

½ cup lower-sodium marinara sauce

1. Preheat the oven to 375°F. Coat a loaf pan with cooking spray.

2. In a large bowl, mix together the turkey, onion, garlic, eggs, bread crumbs, parsley, Dijon mustard, Italian seasoning, salt, and black pepper until thoroughly combined.

3. Transfer the mixture to the loaf pan. Sprinkle the mozzarella cheese and spread the marinara sauce on top. Bake for 45 to 50 minutes, until the internal temperature reaches 165°F.

4. Let slightly cool, then slice into 8 pieces.

5. For leftovers, store in microwaveable airtight containers and microwave on high for 2 to 3 minutes, until heated through.

SUBSTITUTION TIP: For a gluten-free version, use gluten-free panko bread crumbs and carefully read labels to ensure other ingredients are gluten free.

COOKING TIP: Make mini meat loaves by spooning the mixture into greased muffin tin wells. Bake for 15 to 25 minutes, until cooked through.

VARIATION TIP: Try lean ground beef, pork, or chicken.

MAKE IT A MEAL: Try serving with Lemony Green Beans with Almonds (page 197) or Fennel & Grape Potato Salad with Tarragon Dressing (page 200).

PER SERVING: Total Calories: 206; Total Fat: 9g; Saturated Fat: 3g; Cholesterol: 116mg; Sodium: 413mg; Potassium: 39mg; Total Carbohydrate: 9g; Fiber: 1g; Sugars: 1g; Protein: 20g

Turkey & Rice–Stuffed Cabbage Rolls

MEAL-IN-ONE

SERVES 6   PREP TIME: 20 MINUTES   COOK TIME: 1 HOUR 15 MINUTES

Stuffed cabbage rolls are a family favorite probably because one hearty batch can feed a crowd. The cabbage leaves, filling, and tomato sauce can be prepped or the whole dish can be baked in advance and reheated for lunch or dinner. The brown rice and tomato sauce provide fiber while the turkey provides protein for a satisfying meal.

FOR THE TOMATO SAUCE:

1 tablespoon canola oil

½ yellow onion, peeled and diced

3 garlic cloves, peeled and minced

½ tablespoon Italian seasoning

1 teaspoon dried oregano leaves

¼ teaspoon kosher or sea salt

¼ teaspoon ground black pepper

1 (32-ounce) can no-salt-added crushed tomatoes

1 teaspoon granulated sugar

FOR THE CABBAGE ROLLS:

12 cabbage leaves

1½ pounds ground turkey

1 cup Fluffy Brown Rice (page 223)

½ yellow onion, peeled and minced

4 garlic cloves, peeled and minced

1 large egg

1 tablespoon Dijon mustard

2 teaspoons Italian seasoning

½ teaspoon kosher or sea salt

½ teaspoon ground black pepper

½ teaspoon smoked paprika

Preheat the oven to 375°F. Coat a 9-by-13-inch baking dish with cooking spray. Bring a large pot of water to a boil.

TO MAKE THE TOMATO SAUCE:

In a separate Dutch oven or small pot, heat the canola oil over medium heat. Add the onion and sauté for 3 to 4 minutes, until the onion starts to soften. Stir in the garlic, Italian seasoning, oregano, salt, and black pepper. Stir for 30 to 60 seconds so it becomes fragrant. Add the crushed tomatoes and sugar. Bring the sauce to a simmer while you prep the cabbage leaves.

TO MAKE THE CABBAGE ROLLS:

1. Add the cabbage leaves to the boiling water and cook for 2 to 3 minutes, until just wilted. Use tongs to remove them from the water and put them on a cutting board.

2. In a bowl, mix together the ground turkey, rice, onion, garlic, egg, Dijon mustard, Italian seasoning, salt, black pepper, and smoked paprika. Evenly distribute the mixture into the center of each cabbage leaf and roll like a burrito: beginning with the cut end roll the leaf over the filling and then tuck the ends under. Place them in the prepared baking dish, seam-side down. Pour the tomato sauce around the cabbage leaves. Cover with aluminum foil and bake for 30 to 35 minutes. Remove the foil and bake for an additional 20 minutes. Let slightly cool before serving.

3. For leftovers, place the stuffed cabbage rolls in microwaveable airtight containers for up to 5 days. Reheat in the microwave on high for 2 to 3 minutes, until heated through.

SUBSTITUTION TIP: For an even quicker version, use a lower-sodium premade marinara instead of making your own sauce.

COOKING TIP: Cook a large batch of Fluffy Brown Rice (page 223) on the weekend and use in recipes throughout the week.

VARIATION TIP: Try lean ground beef or pork instead of turkey.

PER SERVING: Total Calories: 309; Total Fat: 12g; Saturated Fat: 3g; Cholesterol: 115mg; Sodium: 522mg; Potassium: 201mg; Total Carbohydrate: 22g; Fiber: 6g; Sugars: 9g; Protein: 25g

Creamy Stovetop Turkey Tetrazzini

SERVES 8   PREP TIME: 15 MINUTES   COOK TIME: 30 MINUTES

Tetrazzini is a traditional pasta casserole with mushrooms and peas. This version is lightened up with evaporated milk and stock instead of cream, but it is loaded with flavor from the celery salt, dry mustard, and Parmesan cheese. While typically baked like a casserole, you can make it on the stovetop for a quick weeknight meal.

12 ounces whole-grain spaghetti

2 tablespoons canola oil

1 pound boneless skinless turkey breast, cubed

2 cups sliced mushrooms

1 cup frozen spring peas

3 tablespoons all-purpose flour

1 cup unsalted chicken stock

½ cup low-fat evaporated milk

Zest and juice of 1 lemon

1 teaspoon coarse salt

¾ teaspoon ground black pepper

¼ teaspoon celery salt

¼ teaspoon dry mustard

¼ cup freshly grated Parmesan cheese, divided

½ cup fresh flat-leaf Italian parsley, chopped

1. Bring a large pot of water to a boil. Cook the spaghetti according to package directions. Reserve ½ cup of the pasta water and drain the rest.

2. Heat the canola oil in a Dutch oven or large skillet over medium heat. Add the cubed turkey and sauté for 6 to 7 minutes, until the turkey is almost opaque. Stir in the mushrooms and peas and sauté, stirring frequently, for 3 to 4 minutes, until the mushrooms are tender.

3. Stir in the flour to make a roux, then whisk in the stock and reserved pasta water and bring to a simmer for 3 to 4 minutes, until thickened. Whisk in the evaporated milk, lemon zest and juice, salt, black pepper, celery salt, dry mustard, and half of the Parmesan cheese. Remove from the heat and stir in the cooked spaghetti and chopped parsley.

4. Divide into bowls and top with the remaining Parmesan cheese.

SUBSTITUTION TIP: For a vegetarian version, omit the turkey and add another 2 cups of mushrooms.

COOKING TIP: Add a small amount of pasta water to sauces like this one. It thickens and provides a creaminess without excess calories and fat.

VARIATION TIP: Try diced broccoli instead of mushrooms, if you don't care for mushrooms.

MAKE IT A MEAL: Serve with roasted, sautéed, or grilled vegetables for a complete meal.

PER SERVING: Total Calories: 314; Total Fat: 6g; Saturated Fat: 0g; Cholesterol: 35mg; Sodium: 527mg; Potassium: 262mg; Total Carbohydrate: 39g; Fiber: 5g; Sugars: 5g; Protein: 24g

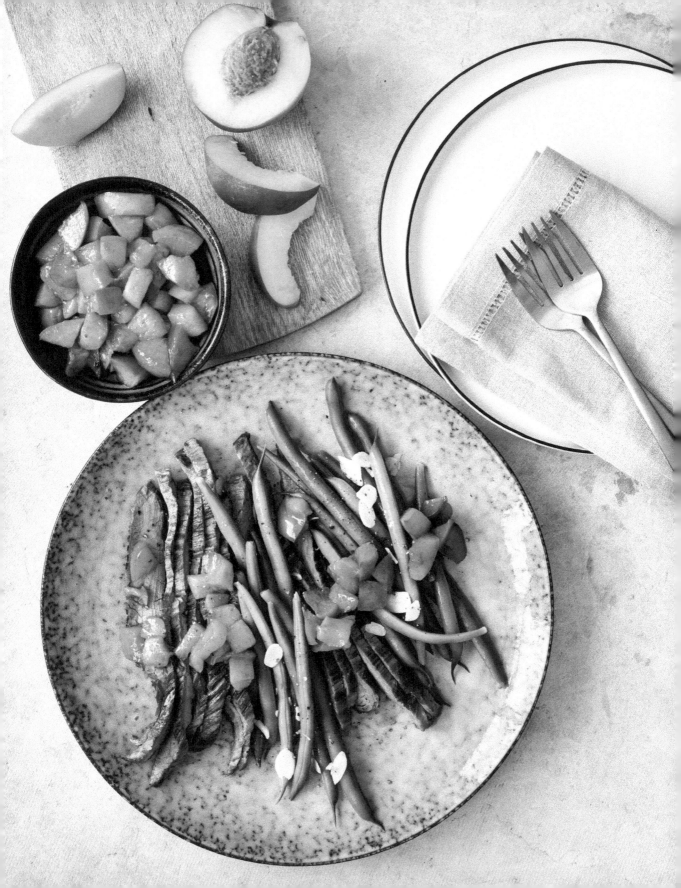

9

Beef and Pork Mains

Grilled Flank Steak with Peach Compote

SERVES 6 PREP TIME: 15 MINUTES COOK TIME: 25 MINUTES

Compote is a simmered, chunky mixture of fruits or vegetables, herbs, and spices—such as cinnamon, ginger, and nutmeg—making it smell like a cheerful winter holiday in your kitchen.

FOR THE PEACH COMPOTE:

2 peaches, cored and diced

1 tablespoon honey

½ tablespoon apple cider vinegar

¼ teaspoon ground cinnamon

¼ teaspoon ground ginger

¼ teaspoon ground nutmeg

¼ teaspoon kosher or sea salt

FOR THE GRILLED FLANK STEAK:

1½ pounds flank steak

2 tablespoons canola oil

½ teaspoon kosher or sea salt

¼ teaspoon ground black pepper

TO MAKE THE PEACH COMPOTE:

Place the peaches, honey, apple cider vinegar, cinnamon, ginger, nutmeg, and salt in a saucepan and bring to a simmer. Stirring frequently, cook for 7 to 10 minutes, until the peaches are tender and the mixture has thickened. Remove from the heat and reserve.

TO MAKE THE GRILLED FLANK STEAK:

Heat a grill or grill pan over medium-high heat. Coat the steak with the canola oil, salt, and black pepper. Grill for 4 to 6 minutes per side, until the internal temperature reaches 155°F. Let rest for 5 to 10 minutes on a cutting board, then thinly slice across the grain. Divide the steak and serve with the peach compote.

SUBSTITUTION TIP: Try maple syrup instead of honey, if desired.

COOKING TIP: Find the grain on the flank steak and slice it against the grain, not with it. If you slice with the grain, the steak will be rubbery and difficult to chew instead of tender.

VARIATION TIP: To give the dish a subtle fall flavor, substitute apples for the peaches when they are in season.

MAKE IT A MEAL: Serve with roasted, sautéed, or grilled vegetables.

PER SERVING: Total Calories: 236; Total Fat: 12g; Saturated Fat: 1g; Cholesterol: 45mg; Sodium: 356mg; Potassium: 69mg; Total Carbohydrate: 7g; Fiber: 1g; Sugars: 5g; Protein: 24g

Beef & Vegetable Stir-Fry

SERVES 4   PREP TIME: 20 MINUTES   COOK TIME: 20 MINUTES

Flank or skirt steaks are the perfect cut of meat for this recipe. They are naturally tender and respond well to quick, dry-heat cooking methods. The broccoli and bell pepper give the dish texture, and the stir-fry sauce, scallions, and sesame seeds round out the flavor.

¾ cup Stir-Fry Sauce (page 222)

2 tablespoons canola oil

1 pound flank or skirt steak, thinly sliced

¼ teaspoon ground black pepper

1 head broccoli, cut into small florets

1 red bell pepper, thinly sliced

1½ cups Fluffy Brown Rice (page 223)

2 scallions, thinly sliced

2 tablespoons sesame seeds

1. Prepare the Stir-Fry Sauce.

2. Heat the canola oil in a large wok or skillet over medium-high heat. Season the steak with the black pepper and cook for 4 minutes, until crispy on the outside and pink on the inside. Remove the steak from the skillet and place the broccoli and peppers in the hot oil. Stir-fry for 4 minutes, stirring or tossing occasionally, until crisp and slightly tender.

3. Place the steak back in the skillet with the vegetables. Pour the stir-fry sauce over the steak and vegetables and let simmer for 3 minutes. Remove from the heat.

4. Serve the stir-fry over rice and top with the scallions and sesame seeds.

5. For leftovers, divide the stir-fry evenly into microwaveable airtight containers and store in the refrigerator for up to 5 days. Reheat in the microwave on high for 2 to 3 minutes, until heated through.

VARIATION TIP: Replace the brown rice with frozen cauliflower rice and follow the preparation directions on the package.

PER SERVING: Total Calories: 408; Total Fat: 18g; Saturated Fat: 4g; Cholesterol: 57mg; Sodium: 461mg; Potassium: 682mg; Total Carbohydrate: 36g; Fiber: 7g; Sugars: 7g; Protein: 31g

Taco-Stuffed Sweet Potatoes

SERVES 4   PREP TIME: 15 MINUTES   COOK TIME: 1 HOUR 20 MINUTES

Sweet potatoes are a great food to eat on the DASH diet. They're loaded with vitamin A, potassium, and fiber, and as an added bonus they provide a sweet quality to savory dishes. For this meal, sweet potatoes are roasted, then stuffed with beef and black bean taco filling and topped with melty cheese and toppings of your choice. It's a winner that everyone will love!

4 small sweet potatoes

1 tablespoon canola oil

½ yellow onion, peeled and diced

1 pound lean ground beef (93% lean)

½ (15-ounce) can no-salt-added black beans, rinsed and drained

2 tablespoons Taco Seasoning (page 216) or store-bought lower-sodium taco seasoning

½ teaspoon kosher or sea salt

½ cup shredded Mexican-style cheese

1 avocado, diced

1 beefsteak tomato, diced

2 scallions, thinly sliced

½ cup fresh or jarred salsa

1. Preheat the oven to 400°F. Poke fork holes in the sweet potatoes, then place them in an aluminum foil–lined baking dish. Roast for 45 to 60 minutes, until fork tender. Let cool, then slice down the center and push back the edges to expose the center of the sweet potato. Turn the oven to a low broil.

2. In a skillet, heat the canola oil to medium. Add the onion and sauté for 4 to 5 minutes, until soft. Add the ground beef and cook for 7 to 8 minutes, breaking up into smaller pieces, until browned. Stir in the black beans, Taco Seasoning, and salt and ½ cup of water. Simmer until the sauce has thickened.

3. Spoon the taco meat into the sweet potatoes and top with the Mexican cheese. Broil for 2 to 3 minutes, until the cheese is melted and bubbly but not burned. Watch them carefully.

4. Top the sweet potatoes with the avocado, tomato, scallions, and salsa.

5. For leftovers, place the stuffed sweet potatoes without toppings in microwaveable airtight containers for up to 5 days. Reheat in the microwave for 2 to 3 minutes, until heated through. Top with the avocado, tomato, scallions, and salsa before serving.

SUBSTITUTION TIP: To make this vegetarian, replace the beef with another can of black or pinto beans.

COOKING TIP: Speed up the process of cooking sweet potatoes by cooking them in the microwave. Select the "potato" button or cook for 7 to 10 minutes on high.

VARIATION TIP: Replace the ground beef with ground turkey or ground chicken.

PER SERVING: Total Calories: 550; Total Fat: 19g; Saturated Fat: 6g; Cholesterol: 80mg; Sodium: 541mg; Potassium: 834mg; Total Carbohydrate: 59g; Fiber: 12g; Sugars: 10g; Protein: 37g

Classic Pot Roast

MEAL-IN-ONE

SERVES 8   PREP TIME: 20 MINUTES   COOK TIME: 3½ TO 4 HOURS

Pot roast is one of those dishes that makes your house feel like home. It's warm, comforting, and satisfying in so many ways. The long cooking process transforms the beef into an extremely tender meal, infused with the flavors of onion, garlic, red wine, and fresh thyme. It can be cooked on the stovetop or in a slow cooker; it's up to you.

2 tablespoons canola oil

2 pounds beef chuck roast

1 teaspoon kosher or sea salt

½ teaspoon ground black pepper

1 large yellow onion, peeled and sliced

4 cloves garlic, peeled

2 cups unsalted beef stock

½ cup dry red wine (optional)

2 bay leaves

5 fresh thyme sprigs

4 Yukon Gold or red potatoes, cubed

2 carrots, peeled and sliced

1. Heat the canola oil in a Dutch oven or stockpot over medium heat. Season the roast with the salt and black pepper. Sear it in the oil for 3 to 4 minutes on all sides, until it has a brown crust.

2. Add the onion and garlic to the pot, then the beef stock and red wine (if using). Bring to a simmer. Add the bay leaves and thyme sprigs. Place the lid on the pot and cook for 3 to 4 hours, until the meat is tender. During the last 30 minutes of the cooking process, add the potatoes and carrots to the pot. Taste and adjust the seasoning, if necessary. Remove the bay leaves and thyme sprigs before serving.

COOKING TIP: For a slow-cooker version, place all ingredients (minus the oil) in a slow cooker with the beef and onions on the bottom and carrots and potatoes on top, for 3 to 4 hours on high or 6 to 8 hours on low, until the beef shreds easily with a fork.

VARIATION TIP: Try adding a few sliced parsnips to the pot roast for an additional potassium boost.

PER SERVING: Total Calories: 320; Total Fat: 12g; Saturated Fat: 3g; Cholesterol: 82mg; Sodium: 430mg; Potassium: 401mg; Total Carbohydrate: 17g; Fiber: 2g; Sugars: 2g; Protein: 33g

Grilled Pork & Pineapple Kebabs

SERVES 6   PREP TIME: 20 MINUTES   COOK TIME: 20 MINUTES

Kebabs are a quintessential summer recipe, and our version got a sweet upgrade with fresh pineapple, red bell pepper, and a mixture of honey, soy sauce, and apple cider vinegar. If you have a bit of extra time, you could marinate the kebabs first, but it's equally delicious brushed on while grilling.

2 pounds pork tenderloin, cubed

1 small pineapple, peeled, cored, and cubed (about 3 cups)

2 red bell peppers, seeded and cut into 2-inch pieces

1 red onion, peeled and cut into 2-inch pieces

¾ teaspoon kosher or sea salt, divided

½ teaspoon ground black pepper, divided

1½ tablespoons canola oil

1 tablespoon honey

½ tablespoon low-sodium soy sauce

½ tablespoon apple cider vinegar

½ tablespoons ground cumin

1. Preheat the grill over medium heat. While the grill is warming up, thread the cubed pork, pineapple, bell peppers, and red onion on skewers, alternating between each ingredient. Season the kebabs with half of the salt and half of the black pepper.

2. In a small bowl, whisk together the canola oil, honey, soy sauce, apple cider vinegar, and cumin and the remaining salt and black pepper. Brush half of the marinade onto the kebabs.

3. Grill for 3 to 4 minutes per side, until the pork reaches 145°F and the vegetables are tender. Each time you flip the kebabs, brush with additional marinade.

SUBSTITUTION TIP: For a vegetarian version, substitute cubed tofu for the pork tenderloin.

COOKING TIP: If using wooden skewers, soak them in water for 30 minutes before threading to avoid them charring or catching on fire.

VARIATION TIP: Try using steak instead of pork and mango instead of pineapple.

MAKE IT A MEAL: Serve with Fluffy Brown Rice (page 223) or Grilled Corn & Edamame Succotash (page 196) to make a complete meal.

PER SERVING: Total Calories: 381; Total Fat: 14g; Saturated Fat: 3g; Cholesterol: 119mg; Sodium: 423mg; Potassium: 844mg; Total Carbohydrate: 17g; Fiber: 2g; Sugars: 11g; Protein: 45g

Slow Cooker Beef Ragu with Creamy Polenta

SERVES 8 PREP TIME: 20 MINUTES COOK TIME: 4 TO 8 HOURS

This delicious recipe is a slow-cooked roast in an onion, garlic, and tomato sauce with a hint of oregano and bay leaf. It can also be braised on the stovetop. The best part is that we pair it with polenta, a creamy, cheesy cornmeal porridge. This hearty recipe is perfect for the winter months. It's hard to believe that it is DASH-friendly.

FOR THE SLOW COOKER BEEF RAGU:

- **2 tablespoons canola oil**
- **2 pounds beef chuck roast, fat trimmed**
- **½ teaspoon kosher or sea salt**
- **½ teaspoon ground black pepper**
- **1 yellow onion, peeled and sliced**
- **4 garlic cloves, peeled and minced**
- **1 (32-ounce) can no-salt-added crushed tomatoes**
- **1 tablespoon dried oregano leaves**
- **2 bay leaves**

FOR THE CREAMY POLENTA:

- **4 cups water or unsalted vegetable or chicken stock**
- **1 cup coarse-ground yellow cornmeal**
- **½ teaspoon kosher or sea salt**
- **1 tablespoon olive oil or unsalted butter**
- **¼ cup freshly grated Parmesan cheese**

TO MAKE THE SLOW COOKER BEEF RAGU:

Heat the canola oil in a large skillet over medium-high heat. Season the chuck roast with the salt and black pepper. Sear the chuck roast in the hot oil for 2 to 3 minutes per side, until a brown crust forms. Transfer the chuck roast to the bowl of a slow cooker. Add the onion, garlic, tomatoes, dried oregano, and bay leaves to the slow cooker. Cook on low for 6 to 8 hours or high for 3 to 4 hours, until the beef shreds easily with a fork. Turn off the slow cooker, discard the bay leaves, and shred all of the beef. Reserve with the lid on until ready to use.

TO MAKE THE CREAMY POLENTA:

1. When the beef ragu has about 30 minutes left to cook, start making the polenta. Place the water or stock in a large saucepan and bring to a boil. Slowly whisk in the cornmeal and reduce the heat to a slow simmer. Cook the polenta for 30 minutes, whisking occasionally, until the liquid has been absorbed and the polenta is creamy.

2. Remove from the heat and whisk in the salt, olive oil or butter, and Parmesan cheese.

3. To serve, add a spoonful of the polenta to a large bowl and top with a hearty scoop of the beef ragu.

4. For leftovers, store in microwaveable airtight containers up to 5 days. Reheat in the microwave on high for 2 to 3 minutes, until heated through.

SUBSTITUTION TIP: Try a pork roast instead of beef.

COOKING TIP: You can also buy instant polenta that cooks in just 5 to 10 minutes.

VARIATION TIP: Try fresh oregano instead of dried and use twice the amount as called for in the recipe for fresh herbs.

PER SERVING: Total Calories: 343; Total Fat: 15g; Saturated Fat: 4g; Cholesterol: 85mg; Sodium: 434mg; Potassium: 344mg; Total Carbohydrate: 19g; Fiber: 3g; Sugars: 4g; Protein: 34g

Chili Garlic-Crusted Pork Chops

SERVES 4 PREP TIME: 10 MINUTES COOK TIME: 15 MINUTES

It doesn't get easier or more delicious than these chili-crusted pork chops. The secret to cooking them perfectly every time is to take the pork chops out of the skillet when they reach 145°F. I love using an instant-read thermometer to do just that. It's also a best practice to let the chops rest for 5 to 10 minutes before slicing to keep the meat tender and juicy.

2 tablespoons canola oil

4 (4-ounce) bone-in or boneless pork chops, trimmed of fat

¼ teaspoon kosher or sea salt

¾ tablespoon Chili Garlic Rub (page 214)

1. Heat the canola oil in a large skillet over medium heat.

2. Coat the pork chops with the salt and Chili Garlic Rub. Cook the pork chops for 3 to 4 minutes per side, until the internal temperature reaches 145°F.

3. Let the pork sit for least 5 minutes before slicing.

SUBSTITUTION TIP: Try boneless skinless chicken breasts instead of pork chops, if desired.

COOKING TIP: Be sure the oil is hot before adding the ingredients to the pan. This will help achieve a golden crust on the pork chops and help them not stick.

VARIATION TIP: Try cooking the chops on the grill for that classic grilled flavor.

MAKE IT A MEAL: Serve with Caramelized Sweet Potato Wedges (page 199) and a side salad for a complete meal.

PER SERVING: Total Calories: 272; Total Fat: 19g; Saturated Fat: 5g; Cholesterol: 66mg; Sodium: 194mg; Potassium: 447mg; Total Carbohydrate: 0g; Fiber: 0g; Sugars: 0g; Protein: 23g

Slow Cooker Pork Carnitas

SERVES 8   PREP TIME: 20 MINUTES   COOK TIME: 3 TO 8 HOURS

Carnitas is slow-cooked juicy pork with hints of onion, garlic, orange, chili powder, and cumin. The meat is typically served with toasted corn tortillas and toppings of your choice. It's a protein-packed meal that is loaded with flavor.

3 pounds pork sirloin roast

2 yellow onions, peeled and cut into wedges

6 garlic cloves, peeled and minced

Zest and juice of 2 large oranges

1 tablespoon chili powder

1 tablespoon ground cumin

¾ teaspoons kosher or sea salt

¾ teaspoon ground black pepper

16 (6-inch) corn tortillas, toasted

½ cup Simple Tomato Salsa (page 211) or store-bought fresh salsa

½ cup fresh cilantro leaves

2 limes, cut into wedges

1. Place the pork roast, onions, garlic, orange zest and juice, chili powder, cumin, salt, and black pepper into a slow cooker. Cook on high for 3 to 4 hours or low for 6 to 8 hours in a slow cooker until the pork shreds easily with a fork.

2. Assemble the tacos by spooning the meat onto toasted corn tortillas and top with the salsa and cilantro leaves. Serve with the fresh lime wedges.

SUBSTITUTION TIP: Try this recipe with a lean beef roast instead of pork.

COOKING TIP: To make this on the stovetop: Heat a tablespoon of oil in a Dutch oven or large pot over medium heat. Sear the pork roast on all sides until browned. Add the onions, garlic, orange zest and juice, chili powder, cumin, salt, and black pepper to the pot, place a lid on top, and braise for 3 to 4 hours, until the pork shreds easily with a fork.

VARIATION TIP: Try Mango Salsa (page 160) instead of the Simple Tomato Salsa or store-bought tomato salsa.

PER SERVING: Total Calories: 368; Total Fat: 10g; Saturated Fat: 3g; Cholesterol: 90mg; Sodium: 405mg; Potassium: 98mg; Total Carbohydrate: 36g; Fiber: 1g; Sugars: 3g; Protein: 31g

Pork Tenderloin with Balsamic Cherry Pan Sauce

SERVES 6   PREP TIME: 10 MINUTES   COOK TIME: 25 MINUTES

Balsamic vinegar and cherries? Believe me, it's an unbeatable flavor combo. In this recipe, pork tenderloin is seared first for a crispy crust, then finished in the oven to ensure that it remains juicy and tender. After removing the meat from the pan, we use the fond—the browned bits of pork that are stuck to the bottom—to make the pan sauce. This gives the sauce an incredible amount of flavor and helps tie it in with the final dish.

2 tablespoons canola oil

2 pounds pork tenderloin

1 teaspoon dried sage

¾ teaspoon kosher or sea salt, divided

½ teaspoon ground black pepper, divided

1 (12-ounce) bag frozen sweet cherries

¾ cup unsalted vegetable or chicken stock

1 tablespoon balsamic vinegar

1 tablespoon maple syrup

1. Preheat the oven to 350°F. Heat the canola oil in a large skillet over medium heat.

2. Rub the pork tenderloin with the sage and half the salt and black pepper. Sear the pork tenderloin in the hot oil for 2 to 3 minutes on each side, until golden brown. Transfer the pork tenderloin to a baking dish and cook in the oven for 15 minutes, until the internal temperature reaches 145°F. Let rest for about 10 minutes, then slice the tenderloin into medallions.

3. Keep the skillet at medium heat and add the cherries, stock, balsamic vinegar, and maple syrup. Let simmer while stirring and scraping the bottom of pan with a wooden spoon for 5 to 6 minutes, until the sauce has thickened and the cherries burst. Season the sauce with the remaining salt and black pepper. Remove the pan from the heat.

4. To serve the pork tenderloin, plate and serve with the cherry pan sauce on the side.

5. For leftovers, store pork tenderloin medallions and cherry sauce in separate microwaveable airtight containers in the refrigerator for up to 5 days. Reheat in the microwave on high for 1 to 2 minutes, until heated through.

SUBSTITUTION TIP: For a vegetarian version, try searing tempeh or seitan and serve it with the balsamic cherry pan sauce.

COOKING TIP: Searing a piece of meat in hot oil then transferring it to the oven to finish cooking is a great way to achieve a brown crust on the outside of the meat with a perfectly cooked center.

VARIATION TIP: Try chopped peaches instead of cherries, if desired.

MAKE IT A MEAL: Serve with Lemony Green Beans with Almonds (page 197) or Maple Mustard Brussels Sprouts with Toasted Walnuts (page 198) for a complete meal.

PER SERVING: Total Calories: 400; Total Fat: 17g; Saturated Fat: 3g; Cholesterol: 119mg; Sodium: 375mg; Potassium: 654mg; Total Carbohydrate: 14g; Fiber: 1g; Sugars: 11g; Protein: 45g

Barbecue Pork Sliders with Avocado Slaw

SERVES 8   PREP TIME: 15 MINUTES   COOK TIME: 3 TO 8 HOURS

Summer cookouts are famous for barbecue dishes, but these sliders are great year-round. The pork is slow cooked for hours until it's fall-apart tender and smothered in homemade tangy barbecue sauce. The avocado slaw can serve as a fresh, crunchy flavorful topping or a side for the sandwiches.

FOR THE PORK:

2 pounds pork sirloin roast

1 cup Carolina Barbecue Sauce (page 219) or store-bought lower-sodium barbecue sauce

FOR THE AVOCADO SLAW:

2 avocados, peeled and pitted

¼ cup nonfat plain Greek yogurt

½ cup fresh cilantro leaves

Zest and juice of 2 limes

1 teaspoon granulated sugar

¼ teaspoon kosher or sea salt

¼ teaspoon ground black pepper

1 (10-ounce) package coleslaw

FOR THE SLIDERS:

8 slider-size whole-wheat sandwich buns

TO MAKE THE PORK:

Place the pork roast in a slow cooker with ¼ cup of water. Cook for 3 to 4 hours on high or 6 to 8 hours on low, until the pork shreds easily with a fork. When cooked, add the barbecue sauce.

TO MAKE THE AVOCADO SLAW:

Place the avocados, yogurt, cilantro, lime zest and juice, sugar, salt, and black pepper in a blender and purée until smooth. Taste and adjust the seasoning, if necessary. Transfer to a large bowl, add the coleslaw, and stir to combine.

TO MAKE THE SLIDERS:

1. Assemble the sliders by spooning the barbecue pork onto slider buns and topping with the avocado slaw.

2. For leftovers, store the pork and slaw in separate containers in the refrigerator for up to 3 to 4 days. Reheat the pork by microwaving on high for 1 to 2 minutes, until heated through. Assemble the sliders right before serving.

SUBSTITUTION TIP: Try a lean beef roast instead of pork, if desired.

COOKING TIP: Adding a small amount of sugar in recipes is not always to sweeten it. Sugar is also a flavor balancer, so we've added it to the avocado dressing to balance the tanginess of the Greek yogurt.

VARIATION TIP: Replace the coleslaw mix with broccoli slaw mix, if desired.

PER SERVING: Total Calories: 364; Total Fat: 13g; Saturated Fat: 3g; Cholesterol: 60mg; Sodium: 545mg; Potassium: 430mg; Total Carbohydrate: 36g; Fiber: 9g; Sugars: 13g; Protein: 28g

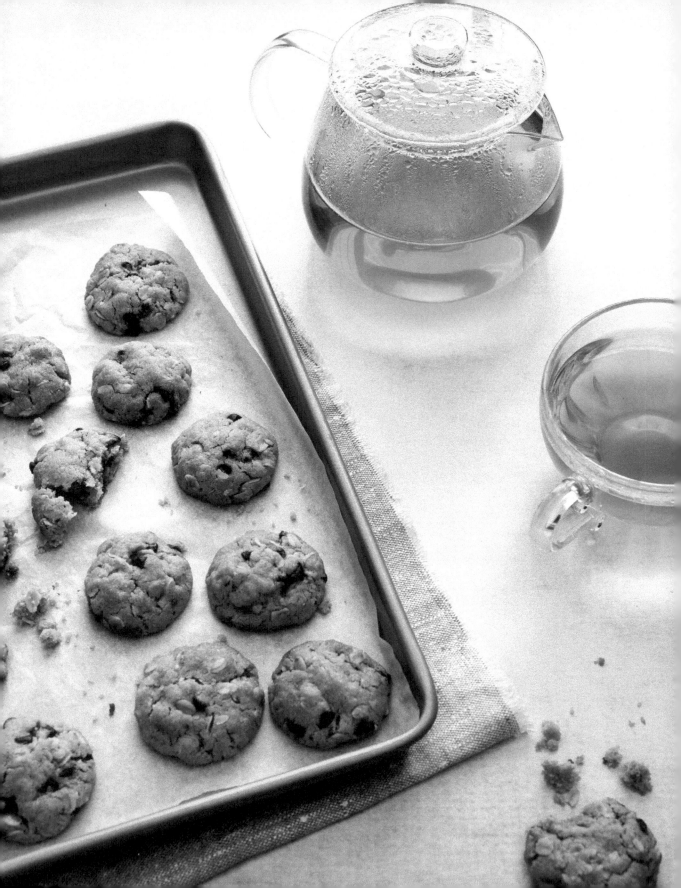

Snacks, Sides, and Desserts

Crispy Cinnamon Apple Chips

VEGAN

SERVES 4   PREP TIME: 15 MINUTES   COOK TIME: 1¼ TO 1½ HOURS

With only four simple and sweet ingredients, these apple chips will become a family favorite. You can use other spices, such as nutmeg, cloves, or ginger, along with cinnamon, if you like. They make the perfect on-the-go or road trip treat.

3 apples, thinly sliced crosswise, seeded

1 tablespoon ground cinnamon

1 teaspoon granulated sugar

¼ teaspoon kosher salt

1. Preheat the oven to 275°F. Coat a baking sheet with cooking spray.

2. In a large bowl, whisk together the cinnamon, sugar, and salt. Add the apple slices and toss to evenly coat. Line up the apple slices on the baking sheet and roast for 45 minutes, then flip each chip and roast for another 45 minutes, until dried and crispy.

3. Once cooled, store in an airtight container or plastic bag for up to 7 days.

SUBSTITUTION TIP: Omit the sugar for an even more DASH-friendly version.

COOKING TIP: It's important to cook these chips low and slow so they can dry out and become crispy without burning.

VARIATION TIP: Try making these chips with pears and dust them with cardamom.

PER SERVING: Total Calories: 80; Total Fat: 0g; Saturated Fat: 0g; Cholesterol: 0mg; Sodium: 147mg; Potassium: 155mg; Total Carbohydrate: 21g; Fiber: 4g; Sugars: 15g; Protein: 0g

Coconut Date Energy Bites

VEGAN · UNDER 30 MINUTES

MAKES 15   PREP TIME: 10 MINUTES

These coconut date morsels are called "energy bites" because of their powerhouse nutrition profile. They contain protein and heart-healthy fats for a satisfying on-the-go snack that is in line with the DASH diet.

12 pitted Medjool dates

½ cup unsweetened shredded coconut

½ cup chopped walnuts or almonds

1½ tablespoons melted coconut oil

Place all the ingredients in a food processor and pulse until the mixture becomes a paste. Form 2-inch bites, place in an airtight container, and store in the refrigerator for up to 2 weeks.

SUBSTITUTION TIP: Add a scoop of protein powder to the mixture, if desired.

COOKING TIP: After processing the mixture, and before forming it into bites, refrigerate it for 30 minutes to make them easier to roll.

VARIATION TIP: Try a variety of mix-ins like oats, peanut butter, mini dark chocolate chips, or raisins to make these energy bites into more of a treat.

PER SERVING: Total Calories: 110; Total Fat: 6g; Saturated Fat: 3g; Cholesterol: 0mg; Sodium: 1mg; Potassium: 151mg; Total Carbohydrate: 16g; Fiber: 2g; Sugars: 13g; Protein: 1g

Roasted Root Vegetable Chips with French Onion Yogurt Dip

SERVES 6 PREP TIME: 20 MINUTES COOK TIME: 20 MINUTES

Consumption of root vegetables may help lower blood pressure. These vegetable chips are baked until golden brown and crispy, and are served with a delicious homemade yogurt dip with caramelized onions, garlic, and seasonings. It is an irresistible and nutritious snack.

FOR THE ROASTED ROOT VEGETABLE CHIPS:

1 sweet potato

1 Yukon Gold potato

1 beet

3 tablespoons canola oil

¼ teaspoon kosher salt

FOR THE FRENCH ONION YOGURT DIP:

1 tablespoon canola oil

1 yellow onion, peeled and thinly sliced

3 cloves garlic, peeled and minced

1 cup nonfat plain Greek yogurt

1 tablespoon mayonnaise

1 teaspoon Worcestershire sauce

½ teaspoon ground black pepper

½ teaspoon onion powder

¼ teaspoon kosher or sea salt

¼ teaspoon dried mustard powder

⅛ teaspoon ground cayenne pepper

TO MAKE THE ROASTED ROOT VEGETABLE CHIPS:

1. Preheat the oven to 425°F. Coat a large baking sheet with cooking spray.

2. Thinly slice the sweet potato, Yukon Gold potato, and beet with a mandoline. Be careful! Coat them in the canola oil and sprinkle with the salt. Roast for about 16 minutes, flipping after 8 minutes, until crispy and lightly browned.

TO MAKE THE FRENCH ONION YOGURT DIP:

1. Heat the canola oil in a skillet over medium-low heat. Add the onion and sauté for 8 to 10 minutes, until caramelized and brown. Stir in the garlic and cook until fragrant, about 1 minute. Transfer the mixture to a bowl and add the Greek yogurt, mayonnaise, Worcestershire sauce, black pepper, onion powder, salt, dried mustard powder, and cayenne pepper. Mix until combined.

2. The chips are best when served immediately. The sauce will keep in the refrigerator for 5 days.

SUBSTITUTION TIP: For a gluten-free version, be sure to buy gluten-free Worcestershire sauce and spices.

COOKING TIP: If you don't have a mandoline, carefully use a chef's knife to thinly slice the root vegetables.

VARIATION TIP: Try making chips out of other root vegetables, like carrots, parsnips, turnips, and rutabaga.

PER SERVING: Total Calories: 168; Total Fat: 11g; Saturated Fat: 1g; Cholesterol: 2mg; Sodium: 266mg; Potassium: 342mg; Total Carbohydrate: 13g; Fiber: 1g; Sugars: 5g; Protein: 5g

Stovetop Cheese Popcorn

VEGAN · UNDER 30 MINUTES

MAKES 15 CUPS   PREP TIME: 10 MINUTES

Nutritional yeast is a popular cheese substitute that is high in vitamin B$_{12}$. Not many plant foods are a great source of vitamin B$_{12}$, making nutritional yeast a popular way for plant-based eaters to get a boost of this energy-boosting nutrient. It's a delicious topping for popcorn and can also be used to make vegan cheese sauce, along with other cheese-flavored dishes.

¼ cup canola oil

½ cup white or yellow popcorn kernels

3 tablespoons nutritional yeast

½ teaspoon kosher salt

Heat the canola oil over medium-high heat in a large stockpot. Add the popcorn kernels and place a lid on the pot. Let cook, shaking the pot periodically, until the popping stops. Remove from the heat, transfer to a large bowl, and top with the nutritional yeast and salt, shaking the bowl to coat the hot popcorn.

SUBSTITUTION TIP: If you can't find nutritional yeast, omit it from the recipe or substitute with freshly grated Parmesan cheese.

COOKING TIP: To make a lower-fat popcorn snack, make popcorn in an air popper instead.

VARIATION TIP: Try spicing up your popcorn with a dusting of chili powder and cayenne pepper.

PER SERVING: Total Calories: 54; Total Fat: 4g; Saturated Fat: 0g; Cholesterol: 0mg; Sodium: 77mg; Potassium: 0mg; Total Carbohydrate: 5g; Fiber: 1g; Sugars: 0g; Protein: 1g

Sweet & Salty Nut Mix

SERVES 6   PREP TIME: 10 MINUTES   COOK TIME: 45 MINUTES

A handful of nuts is filled with heart-healthy fats, protein, and a variety of vitamins and minerals, making them a great snack. Whip up a batch of this sweet and salty mix, and store in bags for a simple snack, ready for any occasion.

1 tablespoon chili powder

½ tablespoon ground cinnamon

½ tablespoon granulated sugar

1 teaspoon ground ginger

½ teaspoon kosher or sea salt

¼ teaspoon ground cayenne pepper (optional)

2 large egg whites

½ cup unsalted peanuts

½ cup unsalted almonds

¼ cup unsalted cashews

1. Preheat the oven to 300°F. Coat a baking sheet with cooking spray.

2. In a small bowl, whisk together the chili powder, cinnamon, sugar, ginger, salt, and cayenne pepper, if using.

3. In a larger bowl, whip the egg whites until slightly frothy. Then, stir in the peanuts, almonds, and cashews. After the peanuts, almonds, and cashews are coated, stir in the spice mixture until combined.

4. Transfer to the baking sheet and spread them out evenly. Bake for 40 to 45 minutes, until slightly browned.

5. Once cooled, store in an airtight container or plastic bag for up to 2 to 3 weeks.

SUBSTITUTION TIP: Use your favorite combination of nuts in this recipe.

COOKING TIP: The egg white is used in this recipe to help the spices stick to the nuts.

VARIATION TIP: For a sweeter version, increase the amount of cinnamon and decrease the amount of chili powder.

PER SERVING: Total Calories: 204; Total Fat: g16; Saturated Fat: 2g; Cholesterol: 0mg; Sodium: 227mg; Potassium: 257mg; Total Carbohydrate: 11g; Fiber: 3g; Sugars: 3g; Protein: 8g

Grilled Corn & Edamame Succotash

SERVES 4   PREP TIME: 10 MINUTES   COOK TIME: 10 MINUTES

Grilling corn on the cob provides depth of flavor and beautiful charring on the kernels. It cooks in about 10 minutes and is a wonderful addition to this edamame, tomato, and fresh herb salad with a light lime vinaigrette. This dish is the perfect accompaniment to grilled meats or fish.

4 ears sweet corn, husked

3 tablespoons olive oil, divided

2 cups shelled edamame

1 pint cherry tomatoes, halved

Zest and juice of 1 lime

¼ cup chopped fresh cilantro

2 tablespoons chopped fresh basil

¼ teaspoon kosher or sea salt

¼ teaspoon ground black pepper

1. Preheat the grill over medium heat. Coat the corn in a teaspoon of the olive oil and grill for about 10 minutes, turning every couple of minutes. Let cool and cut the kernels from the cob.

2. Place the corn kernels, edamame, and cherry tomatoes in a large bowl. Next, add the remaining olive oil, lime zest and juice, cilantro, basil, salt, and black pepper. Stir to combine, and serve with your favorite summer-inspired entrée.

SUBSTITUTION TIP: Try parsley instead of cilantro, if desired.

COOKING TIP: Purchase shelled edamame in the freezer or produce section and let it thaw before adding it to this salad.

VARIATION TIP: Add bell peppers or roasted red peppers, if desired.

MAKE IT A MEAL: Serve with Chili Garlic-Crusted Pork Chops (page 182), Barbecue Pork Sliders with Avocado Slaw (page 186), or Grilled Pork & Pineapple Kebabs (page 179).

PER SERVING: Total Calories: 314; Total Fat: 17g; Saturated Fat: 2g; Cholesterol: 0mg; Sodium: 163mg; Potassium: 432mg; Total Carbohydrate: 32g; Fiber: 10g; Sugars: 6g; Protein: 17g

Lemony Green Beans with Almonds

SERVES 4 PREP TIME: 15 MINUTES   COOK TIME: 15 MINUTES

Green beans are packed with vitamins and minerals, and are low in calories. This recipe dresses them up with olive oil, lemon, Parmesan cheese, and almonds for a delicious side dish.

1 pound green beans, trimmed

2 tablespoons olive oil

Juice and zest of 1 lemon, divided

⅛ teaspoon kosher or sea salt

¼ teaspoon ground black pepper

¼ cup freshly grated Parmesan cheese

¼ cup sliced almonds

1. Bring a large pot of water to a boil. Add the green beans and cook for 2 to 3 minutes. Transfer to a bowl with ice water for 2 to 3 minutes. Drain.

2. Heat olive oil in a large skillet over medium heat. Add the green beans and sauté for 4 to 5 minutes, until lightly browned. Add the lemon juice and simmer for 1 to 2 minutes, then season with the salt and black pepper.

3. Transfer to a serving dish and top with the lemon zest, Parmesan cheese, and almonds.

4. For leftovers, store in microwaveable airtight containers for up to 5 days. Reheat in the microwave on high for 1 to 2 minutes, until heated through.

SUBSTITUTION TIP: For a vegan version, substitute nutritional yeast flakes for the Parmesan cheese.

COOKING TIP: Blanch and shock the green beans, boiling them for a few minutes then transferring them immediately to ice water. This helps keep the green beans crisp and preserves their bright green color.

VARIATION TIP: Try broccoli instead of green beans.

MAKE IT A MEAL: This recipe goes well with a number of recipes from this book including Pork Tenderloin with Balsamic Cherry Pan Sauce (page 184), Crispy Balsamic Chicken Thighs (page 153), Italian-Style Turkey Meat Loaf (page 167), and Spaghetti & Chicken Meatballs (page 159).

PER SERVING: Total Calories: 162; Total Fat: 11g; Saturated Fat: 1g; Cholesterol: 0mg; Sodium: 132mg; Potassium: 294mg; Total Carbohydrate: 10g; Fiber: 5g; Sugars: 4g; Protein: 6g

Maple Mustard Brussels Sprouts with Toasted Walnuts

VEGAN • UNDER 30 MINUTES

SERVES 6   PREP TIME: 15 MINUTES   COOK TIME: 15 MINUTES

Brussels sprouts, a cruciferous vegetable, are a great source of vitamin K, vitamin C, vitamin B$_6$, potassium, and fiber. When sautéed in a hot skillet, they become crispy on the outside and fork tender. The maple mustard sauce and crunchy walnuts take this dish to the next level.

¼ cup chopped walnuts

2 tablespoons olive oil

2 pounds Brussels sprouts, trimmed and halved

¼ teaspoon kosher or sea salt

¼ teaspoon ground black pepper

⅛ teaspoon crushed red pepper flakes

2 tablespoons Dijon mustard

1 tablespoon pure maple syrup

1. Heat a dry skillet over medium heat. Add the walnuts and toast, stirring occasionally, for about 1 to 2 minutes, until lightly toasted. Transfer to a small bowl.

2. Heat the olive oil in the same skillet over medium heat. Add the Brussels sprouts and sauté, stirring occasionally, for 8 to 10 minutes, until slightly fork tender and browned on the outside. Season with the salt, black pepper, and crushed red pepper flakes.

3. In a small bowl, whisk together the Dijon mustard and maple syrup. Pour the mixture into the pan and stir to combine, bringing to a light simmer.

4. Transfer the mixture to the dishes and top with the toasted walnuts.

5. For leftovers, keep the walnuts separate in a small sealed plastic bag and put the Brussels sprouts in microwaveable airtight containers in the refrigerator for up to 3 to 4 days. Reheat in the microwave on high for 1 to 2 minutes, until heated through.

SUBSTITUTION TIP: Try honey instead of maple syrup.

VARIATION TIP: Try broccoli instead of Brussels sprouts.

MAKE IT A MEAL: Serve with Almond-Crusted Tuna Cakes (page 151) or Creamy Stovetop Turkey Tetrazzini (page 170).

PER SERVING: Total Calories: 151; Total Fat: 8g; Saturated Fat: 1g; Cholesterol: 0mg; Sodium: 255mg; Potassium: 611mg; Total Carbohydrate: 16g; Fiber: 6g; Sugars: 6g; Protein: 6g

Caramelized Sweet Potato Wedges

VEGAN

SERVES 4   PREP TIME: 15 MINUTES   COOK TIME: 40 MINUTES

Sweet potato fries are all the rage in restaurants, where they're typically deep fried. Our version features fresh sweet potatoes sliced into wedges, coated in olive oil, and roasted at a high temperature until crispy on the outside and tender on the inside. Serve as a snack or a side dish to make a complete meal.

2 sweet potatoes, cut into ½-inch wedges

2 tablespoons canola oil

¼ teaspoon kosher or sea salt

¼ teaspoon ground black pepper

1. Preheat the oven to 450°F. Line a baking sheet with a wire rack and coat with cooking spray.

2. Evenly coat the sweet potatoes in canola oil and season with the salt and black pepper.

3. Line up the wedges on the wire rack, about 1 inch apart, and roast for 30 to 35 minutes. Turn the oven to a low broil for 3 to 4 minutes, until the edges of the sweet potato wedges are slightly browned. Serve once they have slightly cooled.

4. For leftovers, store in airtight containers in the refrigerator for up to 3 to 4 days. To reheat, line them up on a baking sheet fitted with a wire rack and roast at 450°F for 5 to 6 minutes, until crispy again.

SUBSTITUTION TIP: Try Yukon Gold or red potatoes instead of sweet potatoes.

COOKING TIP: Using a wire rack to bake the sweet potato wedges will help create a crispy crust around the entire wedge.

VARIATION TIP: You can add unique flavors to these wedges by tossing them with a tablespoon of garam masala, Italian seasoning, or chili powder.

MAKE IT A MEAL: Serve these with Chili Garlic-Crusted Pork Chops (page 182) or Grilled Pork & Pineapple Kebabs (page 179).

PER SERVING: Total Calories: 111; Total Fat: 7g; Saturated Fat: 1g; Cholesterol: 0mg; Sodium: 166mg; Potassium: 271mg; Total Carbohydrate: 12g; Fiber: 2g; Sugars: 4g; Protein: 1g

Fennel & Grape Potato Salad with Tarragon Dressing

VEGETARIAN · UNDER 30 MINUTES

SERVES 6   PREP TIME: 20 MINUTES   COOK TIME: 10 MINUTES

Alert: This is not your average potato salad. It has a unique twist. Instead of a mayonnaise-based dressing, this version has a light vinaigrette dressing with fresh tarragon. It also boasts fennel, grapes, and almonds, with a sweet, savory, and nutty touch. Serve it at a party or as a side dish for a weeknight meal.

4 Yukon Gold or red potatoes, cubed

1 small head fennel, cleaned, trimmed, and diced

2 cups red grapes, halved

¼ cup red wine vinegar

1 tablespoon Dijon mustard

1 tablespoon honey

½ teaspoon kosher or sea salt

½ teaspoon ground black pepper

2 tablespoons chopped fresh tarragon

⅓ cup olive oil

¼ cup sliced almonds

1. Bring a large pot of water to a boil. Add the potatoes and cook for 5 to 7 minutes, until slightly tender. Drain, rinse with cold water, drain again, place in a large bowl, and let cool. To the bowl, add the fennel and grapes.

2. In another small bowl, whisk together the red wine vinegar, Dijon mustard, honey, salt, black pepper, tarragon, and olive oil. Add the dressing to the bowl with the salad ingredients and toss to combine.

3. Refrigerate until chilled. Top with the almonds and serve.

4. For leftovers, refrigerate in airtight containers up to 3 days.

SUBSTITUTION TIP: Try chopped walnuts or pine nuts instead of almonds.

COOKING TIP: If using dried herbs, use half the amount as called for in the recipe.

VARIATION TIP: Replace the tarragon with chopped parsley or basil.

MAKE IT A MEAL: Serve with Chili Garlic-Crusted Pork Chops (page 182) or Grilled Flank Steak with Peach Compote (page 174).

PER SERVING: Total Calories: 263; Total Fat: 14g; Saturated Fat: 2g; Cholesterol: 0mg; Sodium: 275mg; Potassium: 707mg; Total Carbohydrate: 33g; Fiber: 3g; Sugars: 13g; Protein: 4g

Grilled Plums with Vanilla Bean Frozen Yogurt

VEGETARIAN · UNDER 30 MINUTES

SERVES 4   PREP TIME: 10 MINUTES   COOK TIME: 15 MINUTES

The grilling process gives this dessert a unique smoky flavor while caramelizing the fruit to make it even sweeter. It's an easy and quick dish that requires very few ingredients, and when served with frozen yogurt and drizzled with cinnamon honey, it'll easily become a crowd favorite.

4 large plums, sliced in half and pitted

1 tablespoon olive oil

1 tablespoon honey

1 teaspoon ground cinnamon

2 cups vanilla bean frozen yogurt

1. Preheat the grill to medium heat.
2. Brush the plum halves with olive oil. Grill, flesh-side down, for 4 to 5 minutes, then flip and cook for another 4 to 5 minutes, until just tender.
3. In a small bowl, whisk together the honey and cinnamon.
4. Scoop the frozen yogurt into 4 bowls. Place 2 plum halves in each bowl and drizzle each with the cinnamon-honey mixture.

SUBSTITUTION TIP: For a vegan option, try dairy-free frozen yogurt and leave out the honey.

COOKING TIP: To achieve perfect grill marks, avoid moving the fruit for those first 4 to 5 minutes.

VARIATION TIP: Try peaches or nectarines instead of plums.

PER SERVING: Total Calories: 192; Total Fat: 8g; Saturated Fat: 3g; Cholesterol: 1mg; Sodium: 63mg; Potassium: 261mg; Total Carbohydrate: 30g; Fiber: 1g; Sugars: 28g; Protein: 3g

Key Lime Cherry "Nice" Cream

SERVES 4   PREP TIME: 10 MINUTES   COOK TIME: 15 MINUTES

"Nice" cream is a trendy version of ice cream that doesn't require cream, nor does it require churning or any special ice cream equipment. The basis of the recipe is frozen banana, and any fruit, citrus, spices, and extracts can be added to give the "nice" cream unique flavors. Simply blend the ingredients in a food processor and enjoy a frozen treat.

4 frozen bananas, peeled

1 cup frozen dark sweet cherries

Zest and juice of 1 lime, divided

½ teaspoon vanilla extract

¼ teaspoon kosher or sea salt

1. Place the bananas, cherries, lime juice, vanilla extract, and salt in a food processor and purée until smooth, scraping the sides as needed.

2. Transfer the "nice" cream to bowls and top with the lime zest.

3. For leftovers, place the "nice" cream in airtight containers and store in the freezer for up to 1 month. Let thaw for 30 minutes, until it reaches a soft-serve ice cream texture.

SUBSTITUTION TIP: You can omit the salt from this recipe if you need to.

COOKING TIP: Peel and slice ripe bananas and place them in a sealed plastic bag before freezing. It is very hard to peel frozen bananas.

VARIATION TIP: Try blueberries and lemon instead of the cherries and lime.

PER SERVING: Total Calories: 150; Total Fat: 0g; Saturated Fat: 0g; Cholesterol: 0mg; Sodium: 147mg; Potassium: 508mg; Total Carbohydrate: 37g; Fiber: 4g; Sugars: 21g; Protein: 2g

Oatmeal Dark Chocolate Chip Peanut Butter Cookies

MAKES 24   PREP TIME: 15 MINUTES   COOK TIME: 10 MINUTES

Our chocolate chip cookies include wholesome ingredients like peanut butter, rolled oats, and dark chocolate chips. Bake them for 8 minutes for a chewier, soft cookie or for 10 minutes for a crispier cookie. The choice is yours. Either way, they make the perfect guilt-free dessert.

1½ cups natural creamy peanut butter

½ cup dark brown sugar

2 large eggs

1 cup old-fashioned rolled oats

1 teaspoon baking soda

½ teaspoon kosher or sea salt

½ cup dark chocolate chips

SUBSTITUTION TIP: For a gluten-free version, choose gluten-free oats.

COOKING TIP: For a fluffier cookie, refrigerate the dough for 30 minutes before baking.

VARIATION TIP: Try raisins instead of the chocolate chips.

1. Preheat the oven to 350°F. Line a baking sheet with parchment paper.
2. In the bowl of a stand mixer fitted with the paddle attachment, whip the peanut butter until very smooth. Continue beating and add the brown sugar, then one egg at a time, until fluffy. Beat in the oats, baking soda, and salt until combined. Fold in the dark chocolate chips.
3. Use a small cookie scoop or teaspoon and place globs of the cookie dough on the baking sheet, about 2 inches apart. Bake for 8 to 10 minutes depending on your preferred level of doneness.

PER SERVING: Total Calories: 152; Total Fat: 10g; Saturated Fat: 3g; Cholesterol: 18mg; Sodium: 131mg; Potassium: 21mg; Total Carbohydrate: 12g; Fiber: 2g; Sugars: 8g; Protein: 4g

Peach Crumble Muffins

MAKES 12   PREP TIME: 25 MINUTES   COOK TIME: 25 MINUTES

The muffin batter is packed with diced peaches, yogurt, and a hint of ginger, and the crumble topping is a sweet mixture of oats and cinnamon. They can serve as a quick breakfast or dessert. They can be made in advance and frozen for future use.

FOR THE CRUMBLE:

2 tablespoons dark brown sugar

1 tablespoon honey

1 teaspoon ground cinnamon

2 tablespoons canola oil

½ cup old-fashioned rolled oats

FOR THE PEACH MUFFINS:

1¾ cups whole-wheat flour or whole-wheat pastry flour

1 teaspoon baking powder

1 teaspoon baking soda

1 teaspoon ground cinnamon

½ teaspoon ground ginger

½ teaspoon kosher or sea salt

¼ cup canola oil

¼ cup dark brown sugar

2 large eggs

1½ teaspoons vanilla extract

¼ cup plain nonfat Greek yogurt

3 peaches, diced (about 1½ cups)

Preheat the oven to 425°F. Line a 12-cup muffin tin with muffin liners and coat with cooking spray.

TO MAKE THE CRUMBLE:

1. In a small bowl, mix together the brown sugar, honey, cinnamon, canola oil, and oats until combined.

TO MAKE THE MUFFINS:

1. In a large bowl, whisk together the flour, baking powder, baking soda, cinnamon, ginger, and salt.

2. In another bowl, use a hand mixer to beat together the canola oil, brown sugar, and one egg at a time, until fluffy. Beat in the vanilla extract and yogurt. Slowly add the flour mixture to the bowl and whisk until the ingredients are just combined. Fold in the diced peaches with a spatula.

3. Fill each muffin well with batter about three-quarters of the way full. Spoon the crumble mixture on top of each. Bake for 5 to 6 minutes, then reduce the oven temperature to 350°F and bake for 15 to 18 additional minutes, until a toothpick inserted into the center comes out clean. Let slightly cool before removing from the muffin tin.

4. Once completely cooled, store in a sealed plastic bag in the refrigerator for up to 5 days or freeze for up to 2 months.

SUBSTITUTION TIP: For a gluten-free version, use gluten-free all-purpose flour instead of whole wheat.

COOKING TIP: When mixing the muffin batter, be sure to mix only until the ingredients are just combined. If the muffin batter is overmixed, it will become tough and dry.

VARIATION TIP: Try blueberries, raspberries, or strawberries instead of the peaches.

PER SERVING: Total Calories: 187; Total Fat: 8g; Saturated Fat: 1g; Cholesterol: 35mg; Sodium: 216mg; Potassium: 100mg; Total Carbohydrate: 26g; Fiber: 3g; Sugars: 10g; Protein: 4g

Peanut Butter Banana Bread Bites

MAKES 24   PREP TIME: 10 MINUTES   COOK TIME: 20 MINUTES

Finding the perfect banana bread recipe can be challenging, but this one is our favorite! That's because it's made into mini bites, so it's easier to control portions yet still has the delicious flavors of bananas and peanut butter. Make them ahead and store in small baggies for a quick and easy snack.

1½ **cups whole-wheat pastry flour**

2 **tablespoons ground flaxseed**

1 **teaspoon baking powder**

½ **teaspoon kosher or sea salt**

½ **teaspoon ground cinnamon**

3 **ripe bananas, peeled**

2 **large eggs**

2 **tablespoons canola oil**

½ **cup dark brown sugar**

2 **tablespoons honey**

½ **cup natural creamy peanut butter**

¼ **cup nonfat Greek yogurt**

1 **teaspoon vanilla extract**

¼ **cup unsalted roasted
   peanuts, crushed**

1. Preheat the oven to 350°F. Coat a 24-cup mini muffin tin with cooking spray.

2. In a bowl, whisk together the flour, flaxseed, baking powder, salt, and cinnamon.

3. In a separate bowl, beat the bananas with a hand mixer set on low. Add the eggs, one at a time, then add the canola oil, brown sugar, and honey. Increase the speed to medium and beat until fluffy. Add the peanut butter, Greek yogurt, and vanilla extract and mix until combined.

4. Reduce the speed to low and slowly beat in the dry ingredient mixture until just combined.

5. Spoon the mixture into each of the muffin wells about three-quarters of the way full. Gently tap the muffin tin on the counter until the batter is evenly spread out. Top with the crushed peanuts.

6. Bake for 20 minutes, until a toothpick inserted into the center of a bite comes out clean. Let rest on the counter until cooled. Remove the bites from the muffin tin.

7. Place in an airtight container or plastic bag and store in the refrigerator for up to 1 week or in the freezer for up to 1 month.

SUBSTITUTION TIP: Replace the peanut butter and peanuts with almond butter and almonds for Almond Butter Banana Bread Bites.

COOKING TIP: If you don't have a mini muffin tin, use a 12-cup muffin tin. Follow the same procedures but cook for 22 to 27 minutes, until a toothpick inserted into the center comes out clean.

PER SERVING: Total Calories: 123; Total Fat: 5g; Saturated Fat: 1g; Cholesterol: 18mg; Sodium: 81mg; Potassium: 96mg; Total Carbohydrate: 17g; Fiber: 2g; Sugars: 8g; Protein: 3g

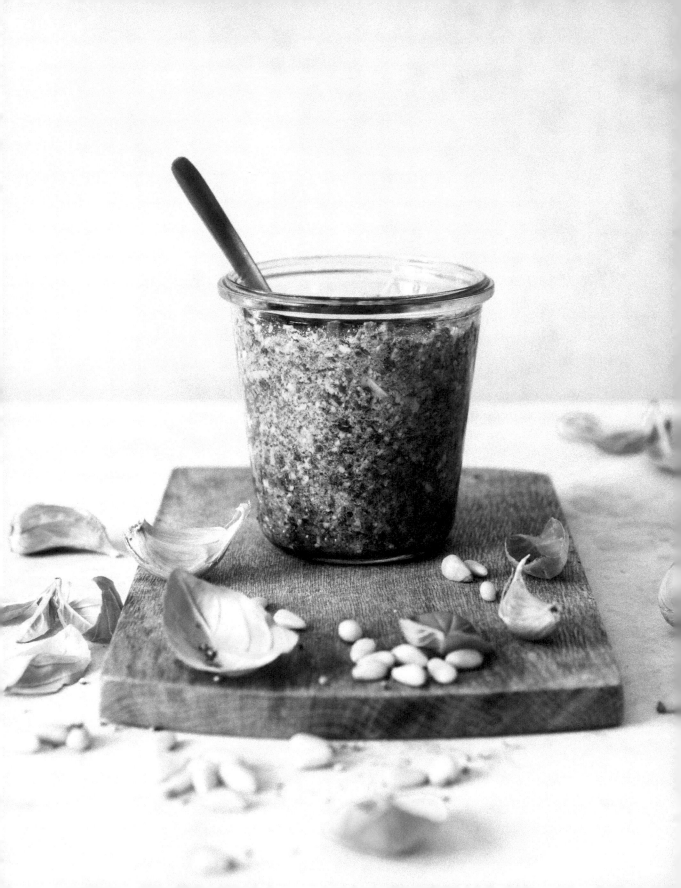

Kitchen Staples, Condiments, and Sauces

Perfectly Poached Eggs

SERVES 4 PREP TIME: 15 MINUTES COOK TIME: 5 MINUTES

Poaching is considered a healthy cooking method because there is no fat required, just water and vinegar. The vinegar helps hold the egg together, so it is essential to add it to the poaching liquid. Poached eggs can also be cooked in advance and reheated throughout the week.

2 teaspoons white vinegar

8 large eggs

1. Pour about a gallon of water into a stockpot and bring to a gentle simmer (160 to 180°F). Stir in the vinegar. Place a few pieces of paper towel on a plate next to you.

2. Stir the water a bit to create a whirlpool. Crack one egg into a small bowl, then slowly slide it into the simmering vinegar water. Repeat this process with the other 7 eggs. Cook for 3 to 5 minutes, until the egg whites are set.

3. Remove the eggs with a slotted spoon and place them on the paper towel–covered plate.

4. For leftovers, place the eggs into a microwaveable airtight container. To reheat, microwave on high for 30 to 60 seconds, until heated through.

SUBSTITUTION TIP: If you don't have white vinegar, use apple cider vinegar.

COOKING TIP: Use an instant-read thermometer to measure the temperature of the poaching water.

PER SERVING: Total Calories: 142; Total Fat: 10g; Saturated Fat: 4g; Cholesterol: 422mg; Sodium: 140mg; Potassium: 0mg; Total Carbohydrate: 0g; Fiber: 0g; Sugars: 0g; Protein: 12g

Simple Tomato Salsa

YIELD: 3 CUPS   PREP TIME: 15 MINUTES

This tomato salsa is made with simple, fresh ingredients and can be customized to fit your preferences. If you don't like spicy foods, omit or reduce the amount of jalapeño. If you're not a cilantro fan, try fresh parsley instead. Tomatillos can also be used instead of tomatoes for a fresh salsa verde.

3 ripe tomatoes, cored and quartered

½ red onion, peeled and quartered

½ jalapeño pepper, seeded

½ cup fresh cilantro

Zest and juice of 2 limes

¼ teaspoon kosher or sea salt

½ teaspoon ground black pepper

½ teaspoon granulated sugar

Place all the ingredients in a food processor and pulse until the desired consistency is reached. Taste and adjust the seasoning, if necessary.

SUBSTITUTION TIP: Omit the jalapeño pepper for a mild version.

COOKING TIP: For a greater depth of flavor, roast the tomatoes with a bit of oil before adding them to the food processor. If you don't have a food processor, finely chop the tomatoes, onion, jalapeño pepper, and cilantro. Toss together in a bowl with the lime, salt, black pepper, and sugar.

PER CUP: Total Calories: 51; Total Fat: 0g; Saturated Fat: 0g; Cholesterol: 0mg; Sodium: 206mg; Potassium: 360mg; Total Carbohydrate: 9g; Fiber: 3g; Sugars: 2g; Protein: 2g

Basil Pesto

VEGETARIAN • UNDER 30 MINUTES

YIELD 3½ CUPS   PREP TIME: 15 MINUTES   COOK TIME: 5 MINUTES

Pesto is a quintessential northern Italian sauce and condiment that features fresh basil. Not only is it delicious, it is considered heart healthy because it's made with superfoods like olive oil, nuts, and garlic. A little goes a long way, though, as it's loaded with flavor but is also calorie-dense.

1 cup fresh basil leaves

1 cup fresh baby spinach leaves

½ cup freshly grated Parmesan cheese

½ cup olive oil

¼ cup pine nuts

4 garlic cloves, peeled

¼ teaspoon kosher or sea salt

¼ teaspoon ground black pepper

SUBSTITUTION TIP: Use nutritional yeast instead of Parmesan cheese to make this recipe vegan.

VARIATION TIP: Try any nuts like pepitas, walnuts, or almonds instead of pine nuts, if desired.

PER ½ CUP: Total Calories: 209; Total Fat: 20g; Saturated Fat: 2g; Cholesterol: 0mg; Sodium: 231mg; Potassium: 65mg; Total Carbohydrate: 2g; Fiber: 1g; Sugars: 0g; Protein: 4g

1. Place all the ingredients in the bowl of a food processor and process until a paste forms, scraping down the sides of the bowl with a spatula as needed. Taste and adjust the seasoning, if necessary.

2. Place leftovers in airtight containers and refrigerate for up to 5 days, or freeze pesto in an airtight container for up to 2 months and thaw as needed. Or divide pesto into cube trays, seal in a plastic bag, and freeze for up to 2 months. Pop pesto cubes out of the ice cube tray as needed.

Chili Lime Marinade

MAKES 2 SERVINGS   PREP TIME: 10 MINUTES

This marinade is perfect for fajitas because the delicious mix of lime, apple cider vinegar, and spices make any cut of meat tender and flavorful. Make it in advance and refrigerate or freeze it to prepare flavor-packed, easy meals any time.

¼ cup canola oil

Zest and juice of 1 lime

2 tablespoons apple cider vinegar

1 tablespoon chili powder

1 teaspoon garlic powder

1 teaspoon onion powder

¼ teaspoon kosher or sea salt

¼ teaspoon ground black pepper

Whisk all the ingredients together, and store in an airtight container in the refrigerator for up to 5 days or freeze it for up to 2 months.

SUBSTITUTION TIP: Try using grapeseed oil or avocado oil, if desired.

COOKING TIP: Marinating imparts a lot of flavor in meats and seafood. However, since it makes the meat wet, it can be difficult to get a crisp sear on the outside unless you dry it off. Once your protein is finished marinating, drain the sauce and pat your protein dry with paper towels before searing.

VARIATION TIP: Use minced fresh garlic instead of the garlic powder, if desired.

PER SERVING: Calories: 266; Total Fat: 27g; Saturated Fat: 4g; Cholesterol: 0mg; Sodium: 291mg; Potassium: 157mg; Total Carbohydrates: 4g; Fiber: 1 g; Sugars: 1g; Protein: 1g.

Chili Garlic Rub

MAKES ABOUT ½ CUP   PREP TIME: 5 MINUTES

Spice rubs are a great way to add flavor to meat, seafood, and vegetables without adding sodium. This version, with savory and smoky notes, is also suitable for adding flavor to Mexican-style recipes. It's a wonderfully versatile rub.

3 tablespoons chili powder

1½ tablespoons garlic powder

1 tablespoon smoked paprika

1 tablespoon onion powder

2 teaspoons ground black pepper

1 teaspoon Mexican oregano or dried
   oregano leaves

¼ teaspoon ground cayenne pepper
   (optional)

Place ingredients in an airtight container or sealed plastic bag and shake to combine. Store for up to 2 months in a dry, dark pantry.

SUBSTITUTION TIP: Try Hungarian paprika instead of smoked if you have it available.

COOKING TIP: Always mix the spice rub in a bowl before patting it on meat, seafood, and vegetables so the spices are equally distributed.

VARIATION TIP: For more spice, add additional cayenne pepper.

PER SERVING: Total Calories: 100; Total Fat: 1g; Saturated Fat: 0g; Cholesterol: 0mg; Sodium: 11mg; Potassium: 440mg; Total Carbohydrate: 22g; Fiber: 6g; Sugars: 1g; Protein: 4g

Garam Masala

VEGAN • UNDER 30 MINUTES

MAKES ABOUT ½ CUP   PREP TIME: 5 MINUTES

Garam masala is a spice mixture common in India and neighboring countries. It can be purchased in the spice section at the grocery store, or you can combine a few common spices to make your own. With hints of warm cinnamon, citrusy and floral cardamom, and spicy black pepper, this spice mixture can be used on or in anything from grilled meats to Indian-style stews and casseroles.

3 tablespoons ground coriander

2 tablespoons ground cardamom

2 tablespoons ground cumin

1 tablespoon ground black pepper

2 teaspoons ground cinnamon

1 teaspoon ground nutmeg

Place the ingredients in an airtight container or sealed plastic bag and shake to combine. Store for up to 2 months in a dry, dark pantry.

SUBSTITUTION TIP: For a spice mixture with greater depth of flavor, use whole pods or seeds, toast them in a dry, hot pan, then grind them with a mortar and pestle or in a spice grinder.

COOKING TIP: When adding herbs and spices to soups, stews, and casseroles, sauté them in the oil before adding any liquid or toast them in a dry, hot pan before use to help release the flavors and create a more flavorful dish.

VARIATION TIP: For a sweeter version, increase the amount of ground cinnamon to 1 tablespoon.

PER SERVING: Total Calories: 156; Total Fat: 5g; Saturated Fat: 1g; Cholesterol: 0mg; Sodium: 30mg; Potassium: 579mg; Total Carbohydrate: 31g; Fiber: 13g; Sugars: 0g; Protein: 6g

Taco Seasoning

MAKES ABOUT ¼ CUP   PREP TIME: 5 MINUTES

Taco seasoning is a staple in most pantries, but so many varieties at your local market are filled with salt and artificial ingredients. It's easy to make a large batch at home, and it can last several months in an airtight container. Our version utilizes smoked paprika and cayenne pepper for a bit of a smoky, spicy kick.

2 tablespoons chili powder

1 tablespoon ground cumin

1 teaspoon smoked paprika

1 teaspoon onion powder

1 teaspoon garlic powder

1 teaspoon Mexican oregano (optional)

½ teaspoon ground black pepper

¼ teaspoon ground cayenne pepper

Combine all the ingredients in a small jar or airtight container and shake to combine. Store in an airtight container for up to 5 days.

SUBSTITUTION TIP: Use dried oregano if you don't have Mexican oregano. Mexican oregano is slightly sweeter and citrusy, but dried oregano will work well, too.

COOKING TIP: Store spices in a dry, dark area such as a pantry to keep them fresher longer. Spices typically last a few months.

VARIATION TIP: Try adding ½ teaspoon of cinnamon for a sweet touch to this taco seasoning.

PER SERVING: Total Calories: 71; Total Fat: 3g; Saturated Fat: 0g; Cholesterol: 0mg; Sodium: 154mg; Potassium: 394mg; Total Carbohydrate: 13g; Fiber: 6g; Sugars: 1g; Protein: 3g

Homemade Chicken Stock

MAKES ABOUT 6 CUPS   PREP TIME: 25 MINUTES   COOK TIME: 3 TO 5 HOURS

Homemade stock is liquid gold. It's filled with fresh flavors and is easily customizable for your cooking needs. This version is made with chicken, but the basic recipe can be modified to make vegetarian, beef, or seafood stock. Just replace the chicken with vegetables, beef bones or meat, or shrimp shells. It can be refrigerated or frozen for future use or used right away to add flavor to any dish.

4 pounds whole chicken or chicken bones

2 onions, quartered

4 carrots, chopped

4 celery stalks, chopped

½ cup fresh parsley stems

4 bay leaves

4 sprigs thyme

2 tablespoons whole peppercorns

1. Pack the chicken or chicken bones, onions, carrots, celery, and parsley stems into a large Dutch oven or stockpot. Cover with cold water and place bay leaves, thyme, and peppercorns on top or in a tied sachet bag. Bring the pot to a low simmer, place the lid on top, and cook for 3 to 5 hours. Discard the bones, chicken fat, vegetables, and parsley stems. Using tongs or a slotted spoon, transfer the chicken meat to a container for future use.

2. Let the stock slightly cool, then strain. Transfer to airtight containers and refrigerate for up to 5 days or freeze for up to 6 months. Before use, skim the fat off the top.

SUBSTITUTION TIP: For a vegetarian version, omit the chicken and double the vegetables in the recipe. Follow the same steps.

COOKING TIP: For a slow cooker version, place all the ingredients in a slow cooker and cook on low for 7 to 8 hours.

VARIATION TIP: Use homemade stock in place of water to make grains, casseroles, soups, and stews even tastier.

PER SERVING: Total Calories: 56; Total Fat: 4g; Saturated Fat: 1g; Cholesterol: 22mg; Sodium: 20mg; Potassium: 54mg; Total Carbohydrate: 0g; Fiber: 0g; Sugars: 0g; Protein: 5g

Homemade Hummus

SERVES 8   PREP TIME: 15 MINUTES

Hummus is a dip or spread made with chickpeas, with origins in the Middle East, where it is still a staple food. There are many variations to the standard recipe, and toppings can be dolloped on top for even more flavor, like olive pesto, roasted red peppers, or garlic and jalapeños. Hummus can be purchased premade at the grocery store, but our homemade version is lower in sodium, without sacrificing flavor. (And it tastes better, too.)

1 (15-ounce) can chickpeas, rinsed and drained

¼ cup tahini (sesame seed paste)

4 garlic cloves, peeled

Zest and juice of 2 lemons

¼ teaspoon kosher or sea salt

¼ teaspoon ground black pepper

¼ to ½ cup olive oil

1. Place all the ingredients in the bowl of a food processor and process until a smooth paste forms, scraping the sides of the bowl with a spatula as needed. Taste and adjust the seasoning, if necessary.

2. Place leftovers in airtight containers and refrigerate for up to 5 days.

SUBSTITUTION TIP: If you can't find tahini at your market, try sunflower butter, or omit the tahini from the recipe for a non-traditional chickpea dip.

COOKING TIP: For a creamier version, use dried beans. Soak garbanzo beans overnight in a bowl of water in the refrigerator, then cook on the stove for about 4 hours, until tender. Skim the shells from the top of the water, drain, and let cool.

VARIATION TIP: Instead of chickpeas, try cannellini beans with Italian seasoning and serve with whole-grain toasted baguette slices. For a Mexican-inspired version, use dark red kidney beans with chili powder and lime, and serve with whole-grain corn tortilla chips.

PER SERVING: Total Calories: 160; Total Fat: 12g; Saturated Fat: 2g; Cholesterol: 0mg; Sodium: 84mg; Potassium: 141mg; Total Carbohydrate: 11g; Fiber: 3g; Sugars: 2g; Protein: 4g

Carolina Barbecue Sauce

MAKES ABOUT 1 CUP PREP TIME: 10 MINUTES COOK TIME: 10 MINUTES

Carolina barbecue sauce is well-known for its tangy flavor from both vinegar and mustard. Although there are thousands of recipes out there, we think ours has the perfect balance of sweet, savory, and spicy. It's also a lower-sodium version of traditional barbecue sauce, made right in your kitchen. So it's DASH-friendly and tasty!

½ **cup apple cider vinegar**

¼ **cup lower-sodium ketchup**

2 **tablespoons brown sugar**

1 **tablespoon honey**

1 **tablespoon yellow mustard**

½ **tablespoon onion powder**

½ **tablespoon garlic powder**

1 **teaspoon chili powder**

½ **teaspoon ground black pepper**

¼ **teaspoon Worcestershire sauce**

1. Add all the ingredients to a saucepan and bring to a simmer. Whisk occasionally until the sauce has thickened, 8 to 10 minutes.

2. Let cool, then transfer to an airtight container and refrigerate for up to 10 days.

SUBSTITUTION TIP: Try maple syrup instead of honey, if desired.

COOKING TIP: Add barbecue sauce to slow-cooked meats for the last 30 minutes of cooking to help impart flavor into the meat.

VARIATION TIP: Replace yellow mustard with Dijon mustard for a unique flavor.

PER ½ CUP: Calories: 136; Total Fat: 0g; Saturated Fat: 0g; Cholesterol: 0mg; Sodium: 120mg; Potassium: 487mg; Total Carbohydrate: 36g; Fiber: 1g; Sugars: 26g; Protein: 1g

Enchilada Sauce

MAKES 6 CUPS   PREP TIME: 10 MINUTES   COOK TIME: 10 MINUTES

Canned enchilada sauce often comes with almost a day's worth of sodium. Making it from scratch is quick, easy, delicious, *and* healthier. Make it ahead and store it in the freezer for a flavor-packed Mexican-inspired sauce anytime.

2 tablespoons canola oil

½ yellow onion, peeled and sliced

5 garlic cloves, peeled and sliced

1½ cups Homemade Chicken Stock (page 217) or store-bought unsalted chicken or vegetable stock

1 (32-ounce) can no-salt-added crushed tomatoes

2 tablespoons chili powder or dried crushed chiles

1 tablespoon ground cumin

¼ teaspoon kosher or sea salt

½ teaspoon ground black pepper

1. Heat the canola oil in a saucepan over medium heat. Add the onion and sauté for 3 to 4 minutes, until soft. Stir in the garlic and sauté for 30 to 60 seconds, until fragrant.

2. Transfer the onion mixture to a blender. Add the stock, crushed tomatoes, chili powder or dried chiles, cumin, salt, and black pepper and purée until smooth.

3. Use the enchilada sauce right away or divide into airtight containers or airtight plastic bags and refrigerate for up to 5 days or freeze for up to 2 months.

SUBSTITUTION TIP: Use no-salt-added tomato sauce instead of crushed tomatoes.

COOKING TIP: If using dried chiles, pay attention to the spice level. Some chiles are hotter than others, so add a little at a time and taste until your desired spice level is achieved.

VARIATION TIP: Try different chiles, such as New Mexico, chipotle, and guajillo, for different spice levels, smokiness, and depth of flavor.

PER SERVING: Total Calories: 96; Total Fat: 5g; Saturated Fat: 0g; Cholesterol: 0mg; Sodium: 118mg; Potassium: 135mg; Total Carbohydrate: 11g; Fiber: 4g; Sugars: 6g; Protein: 3g

Honey Chipotle Sauce

VEGETARIAN · UNDER 30 MINUTES

MAKES ABOUT ½ CUP   PREP TIME: 10 MINUTES   COOK TIME: 15 MINUTES

Similar to barbecue, this honey chipotle sauce has sweet, smoky, and tangy notes, but without copious amounts of salt. Using tomato paste instead of ketchup, which is a traditional ingredient in tangy sauces, helps reduce the sodium levels and provides a rich tomato flavor. The chipotle chiles add heat and smoke flavors, perfectly balancing the honey and vinegar.

1 tablespoon chopped chipotle chiles in adobo sauce

3 tablespoons honey

3 tablespoons no-salt-added tomato paste

3 tablespoons unsalted vegetable or chicken stock

2½ tablespoons white wine vinegar

1. Pour all the ingredients into a small saucepan and bring to a simmer for about 15 minutes, until slightly thickened.

2. Store in an airtight container in the refrigerator for up to 7 days.

SUBSTITUTION TIP: For a vegan version, use pure maple syrup instead of honey and vegetable stock instead of chicken stock.

COOKING TIP: For a smoother version, purée all ingredients in a blender before simmering on the stove.

VARIATION TIP: Try apple cider vinegar instead of white wine, if desired.

PER ¼ CUP: Calories: 136; Total Fat: 0g; Saturated Fat: 0g; Cholesterol: 0mg; Sodium: 124mg; Potassium: 348mg; Total Carbohydrate: 32g; Fiber: 2g; Sugars: 30g; Protein: 1g

Stir-Fry Sauce

MAKES ABOUT 1 CUP   PREP TIME: 20 MINUTES

Stir-fry sauce can be whipped up in a matter of minutes and stored in the fridge to be used all week. It's perfectly balanced, with savory, sweet, umami, and spicy notes. It is used in recipes like Tofu & Green Bean Stir-Fry (page 125) and Beef & Vegetable Stir-Fry (page 175), but can go great with any DASH-friendly stir-fry you want to make.

¼ cup unsalted vegetable, chicken, or beef stock

3 tablespoons low-sodium soy sauce

1 tablespoon honey or brown sugar

2 teaspoons sesame oil

1 teaspoon sriracha (optional)

4 garlic cloves, peeled and minced

1-inch piece fresh ginger, peeled and minced

1 tablespoon cornstarch

In a bowl, whisk the ingredients together until combined. Store in an airtight container in the refrigerator for up to 5 days.

SUBSTITUTION TIP: For a gluten-free version, use tamari instead of soy sauce, and carefully read the ingredient labels to be sure it is indeed gluten free.

PER ¼ CUP: Total Calories: 57; Total Fat: 2g; Saturated Fat: 0g; Cholesterol: 0mg; Sodium: 447mg; Potassium: 17mg; Total Carbohydrate: 8g; Fiber: 0g; Sugars: 4g; Protein: 1g

Fluffy Brown Rice

SERVES 4   PREP TIME: 5 MINUTES   COOK TIME: 50 MINUTES

Brown rice is easily made on the stovetop but can also be made in a rice cooker. There are many varieties of brown rice, such as long grain, basmati, or jasmine, and any will work for this recipe. It just depends on your preference.

1 cup brown rice

2½ cups vegetable stock or water

⅛ teaspoon kosher or sea salt

1. Add rice and vegetable stock or water to a saucepan and bring to a simmer. Place the lid on top and let simmer for 50 minutes, until the water has been absorbed and the rice is tender.

2. Season with the salt and fluff with a fork.

3. Place in airtight containers and refrigerate for up to 3 days.

COOKING TIP: When cooking rice and grains, always read the package directions for the proper cooking liquid ratio and cooking time.

VARIATION TIP: Try any ancient grain, such as quinoa or farro.

PER SERVING: Total Calories: 172; Total Fat: 1g; Saturated Fat: 0g; Cholesterol: 0mg; Sodium: 199mg; Potassium: 100mg; Total Carbohydrate: 36g; Fiber: 2g; Sugars: 1g; Protein: 5g

Honey Whole-Wheat Bread

VEGETARIAN

MAKES 2 LOAVES   PREP TIME: 40 MINUTES PLUS 2 HOURS REST TIME   COOK TIME: 30 MINUTES

Many store-bought loaves of bread are high in sodium, so it's important to read the nutrition labels and compare sodium amounts. This homemade version is simple to make, lower in sodium, and 100 percent whole grain. It can be made in advance and frozen.

1 cup warm water

2 tablespoons honey

4½ teaspoons (2 packets)
   instant yeast

5¾ cups whole-wheat flour or whole-
   wheat pastry flour, divided

½ tablespoon kosher or sea salt

1¼ cups warm low-fat milk

2 tablespoons olive oil

1. In the bowl of a stand mixer, whisk together 1 cup of warm water, the honey, and the instant yeast. Let sit for 5 to 10 minutes, until the mixture is frothy.

2. Add half of the flour to the mixture and whisk to combine. Let sit for 30 to 40 minutes, until foamy.

3. Place the dough hook on the stand mixer. While running on low, slowly add the remaining flour and the salt, milk, and olive oil, then let it run for about 5 minutes, until the dough sticks to the hook.

4. Separate the dough into two balls and transfer to 2 greased loaf pans. Place damp rags over the top of the dough and let it sit for about an hour, until the dough has doubled in size.

5. Preheat the oven to 350°F. Bake for 30 minutes. Let cool, then remove from the loaf pans. Once completely cooled, slice or store whole. Store in sealed plastic bags in the refrigerator for up to 2 weeks or the freezer for up to 3 to 4 months.

SUBSTITUTION TIP: For a vegan version, replace the honey with granulated sugar and the milk with more warm water.

COOKING TIP: When the bread comes out of the oven, brush it with a small amount of olive oil.

VARIATION TIP: To increase the soluble fiber content in this bread, instead of all whole-wheat flour, use a mix of equal parts oat flour and whole-wheat flour.

PER SLICE: Total Calories: 94; Total Fat: 1g; Saturated Fat: 0g; Cholesterol: 0mg; Sodium: 114mg; Potassium: 1mg; Total Carbohydrate: 18g; Fiber: 46g; Sugars: 3g; Protein: 2g

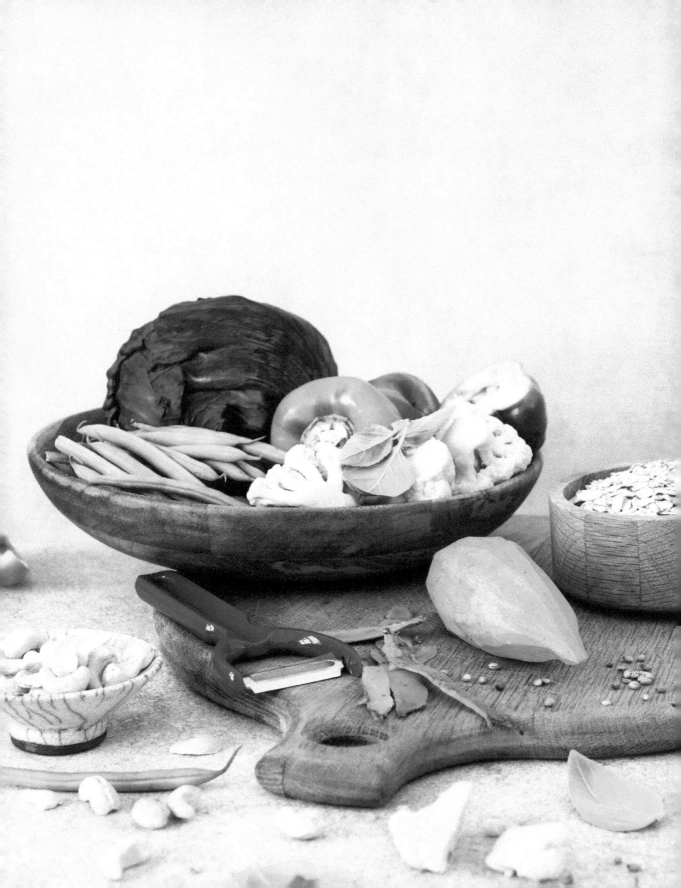

Measurement Conversions

VOLUME EQUIVALENTS (LIQUID)

US STANDARD	US STANDARD (OUNCES)	METRIC (APPROXIMATE)
2 tablespoons	1 fl. oz.	30 mL
¼ cup	2 fl. oz.	60 mL
½ cup	4 fl. oz.	120 mL
1 cup	8 fl. oz.	240 mL
1½ cups	12 fl. oz.	355 mL
2 cups or 1 pint	16 fl. oz.	475 mL
4 cups or 1 quart	32 fl. oz.	1 L
1 gallon	128 fl. oz.	4 L

OVEN TEMPERATURES

FAHRENHEIT	CELSIUS (APPROXIMATE)
250°F	120°C
300°F	150°C
325°F	165°C
350°F	180°C
375°F	190°C
400°F	200°C
425°F	220°C
450°F	230°C

VOLUME EQUIVALENTS (DRY)

US STANDARD	METRIC (APPROXIMATE)
⅛ teaspoon	0.5 mL
¼ teaspoon	1 mL
½ teaspoon	2 mL
¾ teaspoon	4 mL
1 teaspoon	5 mL
1 tablespoon	15 mL
¼ cup	59 mL
⅓ cup	79 mL
½ cup	118 mL
⅔ cup	156 mL
¾ cup	177 mL
1 cup	235 mL
2 cups or 1 pint	475 mL
3 cups	700 mL
4 cups or 1 quart	1 L

WEIGHT EQUIVALENTS

US STANDARD	METRIC (APPROXIMATE)
½ ounce	15 g
1 ounce	30 g
2 ounces	60 g
4 ounces	115 g
8 ounces	225 g
12 ounces	340 g
16 ounces or 1 pound	455 g

References

American Psychological Association. "Stressed in America." Accessed July 7, 2018. http://www.apa.org/monitor/2011/01/stressed-america.aspx.

Appel, Lawrence, Thomas Moore, Eva Obarzanek, William Vollmer, Laura Svetsky, Frank Sacks, George Bray et al. "A Clinical Trial of the Effects of Dietary Patterns on Blood Pressure." *New England Journal of Medicine* 336, no. 16 (1997): 1117–24.

Beccuti, G., and S. Pannain. "Sleep and Obesity." *Current Opinion in Clinical Nutrition and Metabolic Care* 14, no. 4 (July 2011): 402–12.

Block, J. P., Y. He, A. M. Zaslavsky, L. Ding, and J. Z. Ayanian. "Psychosocial Stress and Change in Weight among US Adults." *American Journal of Epidemiology* 170, no. 2 (July 15, 2009): 181–92.

CDC. "Tips for Better Sleep." Accessed September 16, 2018. https://www.cdc.gov /sleep/about_sleep/sleep_hygiene.html.

Centers for Disease Control and Prevention. "National Diabetes Statistics Report, 2017: Estimates of Diabetes and Its Burden on the United States." Accessed July 5, 2018. https://www.cdc.gov/diabetes/pdfs/data/statistics/national-diabetes -statistics-report.pdf.

Chaprut, Jean-Phillipe, Jean-Pierre Despres, Claude Bouchard, and Angelo Tremblay. "The Association between Sleep Duration and Weight Gain in Adults: A 6-Year Prospective Study from the Quebec Family Study." *Sleep* 31, no. 4 (2008): 517–23.

Consensus Conference, Panel, N. F. Watson, M. S. Badr, G. Belenky, D. L. Bliwise, O. M. Buxton, D. Buysse. "Joint Consensus Statement of the American Academy of

Sleep Medicine and Sleep Research Society on the Recommended Amount of Sleep for a Healthy Adult: Methodology and Discussion." *Sleep* 38, no. 8 (August 1, 2015): 1161–83.

Cox, Carla E. "Role of Physical Activity for Weight Loss and Weight Maintenance." *Diabetes Spectrum* 30, no. 3 (2017): 157–60.

Dombrowski, S. U., K. Knittle, A. Avenell, V. Araujo-Soares, and F. F. Sniehotta. "Long Term Maintenance of Weight Loss with Non-Surgical Interventions in Obese Adults: Systematic Review and Meta-Analyses of Randomised Controlled Trials." *BMJ* 348 (May 14, 2014): g2646.

Finkler, E., S. B. Heymsfield, and M. P. St-Onge. "Rate of Weight Loss Can Be Predicted by Patient Characteristics and Intervention Strategies." *Journal of the Academy of Nutrition and Dietetics* 112, no. 1 (January 2012): 75–80.

Gottelieb, D. J., S. Redline, F. J. Nieto, C. M. Baldwin, A. B. Newman, H. E. Resnick, and N. M. Penjabi. "Association of Usual Sleep Duration with Hypertension: The Sleep Heart Health Study." *Sleep* 29, no. 8 (2006): 1009–14.

Hall, Kevin D. "What Is the Required Energy Deficit Per Unit Weight Loss?" *International Journal of Obesity* 32, no. 3 (2008): 573–76.

Kokkinos, P. "Physical Activity, Health Benefits, and Mortality Risk." *ISRN Cardiology* 2012 (2012). https://doi.org/10.5402/2012/718789.

Kondo, M. C., S. F. Jacoby, and E. C. South. "Does Spending Time Outdoors Reduce Stress? A Review of Real-Time Stress Response to Outdoor Environments." *Health Place* 51 (May 2018): 136–50.

Lear, Scott A., Weihong Hu, Sumathy Rangarajan, Danijela Gasevic, Darryl Leong, Romaina Iqbal, Amparo Casanova, et al. "The Effect of Physical Activity on Mortality and Cardiovascular Disease in 130 000 People from 17 High-Income, Middle-Income, and Low-Income Countries: The PURE Study." *The Lancet* 390, no. 10113 (2017): 2643–54.

Leidy, H. J., P. M. Clifton, A. Astrup, T. P. Wycherley, M. S. Westerterp-Plantenga, N. D. Luscombe-Marsh, S. C. Woods, and R. D. Mattes. "The Role of Protein in Weight Loss and Maintenance." *The American Journal of Clinical Nutrition* 101, issue 6 (June 1, 2015): 1320S–1329S. https://doi.org/10.3945/ajcn.114.084038.

Mekary, R. A., A. Grontved, J. P. Despres, L. P. De Moura, M. Asgarzadeh, W. C. Willett, E. B. Rimm, E. Giovannucci, and F. B. Hu. "Weight Training, Aerobic Physical Activities, and Long-Term Waist Circumference Change in Men." *Obesity (Silver Spring)* 23, no. 2 (February 2015): 461–67.

Nwankwo, Tatiana, Sung Sug Yoon, Vicki Burt, and Quiping Gu. "Hypertension among Adults in the United States: National Health and Nutrition Examination Survey, 2011–2012." Accessed September 16, 2018. https://www.cdc.gov/nchs/products/databriefs/db133.htm.

Palagini, Laura, Rosa Maria Bruno, Angelo Gemignani, Chiara Baglioni, Lorenzo Ghiadoni, and Dieter Riemann. "Sleep Loss and Hypertension: A Systematic Review." *Current Pharmaceutical Design* 19, no. 13 (2013): 2409–19.

Presse, Nancy, Sylvie Belleville, Pierrette Gaudreau, Carol E. Greenwood, Marie-Jeanne Kergoat, Jose A. Morais, Hélène Payette, Bryna Shatenstein, and Guylaine Ferland. "Vitamin K Status and Cognitive Function in Healthy Older Adults." *Neurobiology of Aging* 34, no. 12 (2013): 2777–83.

Sacks, Frank, Lawrence Appel, Thomas Moore, Eva Obarzanek, William Vollmer, Laura Svetsky, George Bray, et al. "Effects on Blood Pressure of Reduced Dietary Sodium and the Dietary Approaches to Stop Hypertension (Dash) Diet." *New England Journal of Medicine* 344, no. 1 (2001): 3–10.

Soltani, S., F. Shirani, M. J. Chitsazi, and A. Salehi-Abargouei. "The Effect of Dietary Approaches to Stop Hypertension (Dash) Diet on Weight and Body Composition in Adults: A Systematic Review and Meta-Analysis of Randomized Controlled Clinical Trials." *Obesity Reviews* 17, no. 5 (May 2016): 442–54.

Stavrou, Stavroula, Nicolas Nicolaides, Iflgenia Papageorgiou, Pinelopi Papadopoulou, Elena Terzioglou, George Chrousos, Christina Darviri, and Evangella Charmandari.

"The Effectiveness of a Stress-Management Intervention Program in the Management of Overweight and Obesity in Childhood and Adolescence." *Journal of Molecular Biology* 5, no. 2 (2016): 63–70.

Strasser, B., A. Spreitzer, and P. Haber. "Fat Loss Depends on Energy Deficit Only, Independently of the Method for Weight Loss." *Annals of Nutrition and Metabolism* 51, no. 5 (2007): 428–32.

Swift, D. L., N. M. Johannsen, C. J. Lavie, C. P. Earnest, and T. S. Church. "The Role of Exercise and Physical Activity in Weight Loss and Maintenance." *Progress in Cardiovascular Diseases* 56, no. 4 (January–February 2014): 441–47.

Tucker, L. A., and K. S. Thomas. "Increasing Total Fiber Intake Reduces Risk of Weight and Fat Gains in Women." *The Journal of Nutrition* 139, no. 3 (March 2009): 576–81.

Verheggen, R. J., M. F. Maessen, D. J. Green, A. R. Hermus, M. T. Hopman, and D. H. Thijssen. "A Systematic Review and Meta-Analysis on the Effects of Exercise Training Versus Hypocaloric Diet: Distinct Effects on Body Weight and Visceral Adipose Tissue." *Obesity Reviews* 17, no. 8 (August 2016): 664–90.

World Health Organization. "Part Two. The Urgent Need for Action: Chapter One. Chronic Diseases: Causes and Health Impact." Accessed on July 12, 2018. http://www.who.int/chp/chronic_disease_report/part2_ch1/en.

Recipe Index

Index

Acknowledgments

I have to first thank my small but immensely strong support system including my parents, sister, extended family, and friends. I know many of you will purchase and promote this book purely to support me, and I truly appreciate that.

When I started my journey in private practice and blogging three years ago, I could only have dreamed of becoming a published author. Your belief and support have been instrumental in allowing me to turn my dreams into reality.

This goes for Josh, Nonna Pina, Nonna Maria, Nonno Pepe, and Zio Ferruccio as well. Although you aren't here to share in this achievement, know that I keep you with me always.

—Andy

To my husband, Ben, for indulging me in all my wild and crazy dreams, your willingness to wash seemingly endless dishes, and being the best taste tester anyone could ask for. Your support, humor, and encouragement keep me going every day.

To those who have given me a chance in my career and those who have inspired me, even if we have never met.

And to each and every one of you who had the courage to pick up this book, get in the kitchen, and start cooking: You are my people. I'm so glad we're on this journey together, and I hope you enjoy every morsel of it. This book has connected us through food, cooking, and good health, and for that I am forever grateful.

Never stop cooking.

—Julie

About the Authors

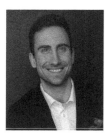 **Andy De Santis, RD, MPH,** is a registered dietitian from Toronto, Canada. He operates a private practice that focuses on customized nutrition solutions and healthy eating. There is nothing he loves more than helping people reach their diet and nutrition goals, and he also holds a master's degree in public health nutrition from the Dalla Lana School of Public Health at the University of Toronto. Before pursuing private practice, Andy was employed at Diabetes Canada. When he isn't helping people in a one-on-one setting, Andy loves offering far-reaching nutrition education through his own personal blog, AndyTheRD.com, and his various social media accounts.

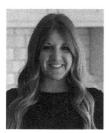 **Julie Andrews, MS, RDN, CD,** is a registered dietitian nutritionist and trained chef with a master's degree in human nutrition. She is the creator and owner of The Gourmet RD, where she is a food and nutrition consultant, cookbook author, recipe developer, food photographer, food and nutrition writer, and culinary media expert. She is regularly featured on television and in the media, where she shares nutrition expertise and showcases simple, wholesome, and delicious recipes from her blog, TheGourmetRD.com. Julie's greatest passion is helping others build confidence in the kitchen and inspiring them to cook for themselves, as she truly believes it's the ticket to better health and a more enjoyable life.

CPSIA information can be obtained
at www.ICGtesting.com
Printed in the USA
BVHW091052091118
532664BV00019B/875/P

9 781641 521390